Exercise and Young People

Exercise and Young People

Issues, Implications and Initiatives

Edited by

Lorraine Cale

and

Jo Harris

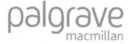

First published 2005 by
PALGRAVE MACMILLAN
Houndmills, Basingstoke, Hampshire RG21 6XS and
175 Fifth Avenue, New York, N.Y. 10010
Companies and representatives throughout the world

PALGRAVE MACMILLAN is the global academic imprint of the Palgrave
Macmillan division of St. Martin's Press, LLC and of Palgrave Macmillan Ltd.
Macmillan® is a registered trademark in the United States, United Kingdom
and other countries. Palgrave is a registered trademark in the European
Union and other countries.

ISBN 1–4039–0252–6

This book is printed on paper suitable for recycling and made from fully
managed and sustained forest sources.

A catalogue record for this book is available from the British Library.

10 9 8 7 6 5 4 3 2 1
14 13 12 11 10 09 08 07 06 05

Printed and bound in China

Contents

List of Figures

List of Tables

Acknowledgements

We would like to thank Magenta Lampson and Jon Reed for their support and advice throughout the preparation of this text.

We are also grateful to the following for their kind permission to use the specified figures and tables: Human Kinetics, Champaign, IL (Figure 3.1); Terry Graham (Editor-in-Chief, Canadian Journal of Applied Physiology), Human Biology and Nutritional Sciences, University of Guelph, Guelph, Ontario, Canada (Figure 3.2); Lippincott Williams & Wilkins, Philadelphia, PA (Table 4.1); Human Kinetics Europe Ltd (Tables 5.4 and 7.1); MCB University Press (Table 5.5); the Physical Education Association of the United Kingdom (Figure 7.1; Tables 9.2 and 9.3).

Every effort has been made to contact all copyright holders, but if any have been inadvertently omitted, the publishers will be pleased to make the necessary arrangements at the earliest opportunity.

Notes on Contributors

Lorraine Cale is a senior lecturer in the School of Sport and Exercise Sciences and Director of PE Teacher Education at Loughborough University. Her research interests include exercise and young people, and particularly physical activity promotion in schools, within and beyond the curriculum.

Trish Gorely is a lecturer in physical activity and health in the School of Sport and Exercise Sciences at Loughborough University. She studied physical education at Otago University, New Zealand before gaining an M.Ed. and Ph.D. in sport and exercise psychology from the University of Western Australia. Her main research interests are in understanding physical inactivity and factors influencing the adoption of active lifestyles.

Jo Harris is a senior lecturer in the School of Sport and Exercise Sciences and Director of Teacher Education at Loughborough University. She is also President of the Physical Education Association of the UK. She is actively involved in research studying health-related policy and practice within the curriculum.

Jim McKenna is a senior lecturer and Director of MSc Studies in the Department of Exercise and Health Sciences at the University of Bristol. His research interests range from counselling for behaviour change in exercise, nutrition and injury rehabilitation to exercise in the elderly.

Chris Riddoch, at the time of writing, was a senior lecturer in the Department of Exercise and Health Sciences at the University of Bristol. He is now Head of the Institute for Sport and Exercise at Middlesex University. His research interests include children's health and fitness and physical activity promotion.

1

Young People and Exercise – Introduction and Overview

Lorraine Cale and Jo Harris

> Children are one third of our population and all of our future. (Select
> Panel for the Promotion of Child Health, 1981)

The purpose of this chapter is to provide a rationale, case for and general
chapter-by-chapter overview of this book, as well as to introduce the terms
and concepts that are central to the area of young people, exercise and
health.

About the book

The notion that young people are not as active, fit and healthy as they
should be is not new and has attracted widespread interest from
researchers, government, health practitioners, educationalists and the
media in recent years. Some have gone so far as to label the youth of
today as 'couch kids', and have referred to current concerns over young
people's inactivity as a 'growing epidemic'. Similarly, the view that there
are links between childhood physical activity and childhood and adult
health, childhood activity and activity in adulthood, and between childhood activity and other health behaviours has become increasingly
attractive. In other words, active children are more likely to be healthier
(as children and adults), become active adults, and are also more likely
to be non-smokers, eat more healthily, and so on.

One only has to observe the lifestyle and habits of Harry Enfield's 'infamous' teenage character, Kevin, to appreciate the concerns about today's youth. Kevin is addicted to TV, computer games, labour-saving gadgets and junk food. He is, furthermore, taxied everywhere by his devoted parents and will go to great lengths to escape active chores such as tidying his room or washing the car! He does of course, like most young people, own a pair of trainers, but these are evidently merely a fashion accessory – their only wear and tear comes from being dragged along the floor as he walks. Yes, even picking up his feet is too much of a physical effort for the tiresome teenager. Whilst it might be argued that many of these behaviours simply depict those of a 'typical' teenager from any generation, there is no doubt that the pressures upon and the opportunities for Kevin, as a young person growing up in today's society, to be sedentary are immense. Chapter 8 explores such pressures in some detail.

Surprisingly though, although we might all recognize the above and anecdotally have experiences and examples which we could share to illustrate how inactive, unfit and unhealthy today's youth are, there is little empirical evidence to confirm this picture. In contrast to adults, and as Chapter 2 highlights, the evidence base for young people is still relatively weak and there continues to be debate about the nature and extent of the problem and the range of possible solutions.

Broadly, this book aims to enhance our understanding of exercise and young people. Based on the evidence available on young people's physical activity and physical fitness, and their influence on health, the book explores the key issues, implications and initiatives associated with exercise and physical activity promotion in young people. Young people are a distinct group with specific health and physical activity needs. Despite this, however, and perhaps as a result of the limited evidence available, there appear to be a number of myths, misconceptions and confusions, and a general lack of guidance concerning young people's physical activity and fitness, and the promotion of physical activity in particular. Given this, the book draws together the available evidence to establish what precisely is known about young people's physical activity and fitness, and then explores the key issues and the implications of these facts for physical activity promotion practice. Indeed, 'application to practice' is a major and important focus of the book. In short, we hope that the book will provide a greater insight into some of the following important questions in the field:

- How important is physical activity to young people's health?
- How physically active and fit are young people?
- How do we measure young people's physical activity and physical fitness?
- How much physical activity should young people do?
- What factors influence young people's physical activity behaviour?
- How can schools and communities promote physical activity to young people?
- How effective are school and community-based physical activity interventions?
- What initiatives, strategies, resources and contacts are available to support the promotion of physical activity in young people?

In addition, the book explores many of the contentious and debated issues associated with the promotion of physical activity in young people, such as fitness testing and the application of physical activity guidelines to young people, again providing guidance and recommendations for practice.

We hope that the area and the focus of the book, on both theory and practice, will appeal to and satisfy the needs of undergraduate and post-graduate students studying physical education, sport or exercise science related courses, as well as physical education, sport and health practitioners (e.g. physical education teachers, school sport co-ordinators, health/exercise promotion officers, sports development officers, coaches) and others involved in working with young people (e.g. youth/community workers). Because the book is intended for a wide range of individuals and groups, interspersed through the text are a number of interactive activities, discussion points and case studies which we hope reflect the diversity of needs and interests. These aim to encourage reflection and debate and, where applicable, to enable the reader to apply the knowledge and understanding to their own practice.

Chapter-by-chapter overview

Following on from this introductory chapter, Chapter 2 explores the current evidence on young people's physical activity and fitness status and the association between physical activity, fitness, and current and future health. The evidence concerning the relationship between activity, fitness and health is reviewed with respect to various health outcomes and young people's physical activity is explored with respect to their overall activity levels, patterns and habits. The consideration of young people's physical fitness is restricted to aerobic fitness (as measured in the laboratory) primarily because of its relationship to specific 'health' or disease outcomes. The key findings and issues concerning young people's physical activity and aerobic fitness are summarized, and consistent trends in the data are highlighted.

Chapter 3 considers the purposes and methods of monitoring physical fitness and physical activity in young people and the relative strengths and limitations of the different approaches. Particular attention is afforded to monitoring physical activity and the practical application of physical activity assessments. As explained, this emphasis reflects the public health and physical activity promotion perspective of this book, as well as current thinking in the area which has called for a shift away from the 'product' of physical fitness and physical fitness testing, towards the 'process' of being physically active and the promotion of physical activity.

If we are successfully to promote physical activity in young people, we need to understand why some young people are active and others are not. Chapter 4 uses an ecological perspective to structure a discussion of the determinants or correlates of physical activity in young people, and how this information can be used in applied settings. In addition, and more recently in response to calls to study sedentary behaviour as a concept distinct from physical activity, the chapter discusses the determinants of some of the most prevalent sedentary behaviours. This is based on the rationale that, by identifying consistent determinants of sedentary behaviours, more effective interventions to reduce them may be possible, resulting in increases in physical activity.

A particular area of interest is how much physical activity young people should do, and how much is enough? These questions are addressed in Chapter 5 which explores the major developments in exercise recommendations for young people in recent years. A brief historical overview of exercise recommendations for young people is provided but the chapter focuses primarily on the most recent UK guidelines which have been developed for England (HEA, 1998) and Scotland (Scottish Executive, 2003). The background, nature, evidence and rationale for the recommendations are considered and their value and practical application discussed. Ideas as to how they can be implemented by physical educators, health and other professionals in the promotion of physical activity are presented, as well as some general cautions and key messages concerning their implementation.

Having reviewed the evidence base surrounding young people's physical activity and fitness, and the factors influencing such status, the latter chapters in the book are concerned with how we might address these issues via effective physical activity promotion practice. Chapter 6 considers the different theoretical approaches and models of exercise or physical activity behaviour change available (from psychological to social theories). The key components and theoretical features of the dominant models are explored and a range of the contemporary theoretical and practical concerns are addressed. By so doing, the chapter aims to highlight useful opportunities for innovative developments in both theory and practice.

Chapters 7 and 8 explore the promotion of physical activity in young people within two key contexts, the school and the community, and consider their role, their potential and some of the major issues and considerations for promoting activity within both contexts. The former chapter advocates a whole-school approach and philosophy to the promotion of physical activity and health, and explores the concepts and characteristics of a 'healthy' and 'active' school. The many avenues through which physical activity can be promoted within the school are highlighted, and particular attention is paid to the promotion of physical activity through the PE curriculum. An analysis and discussion of the key issues and debates concerning meeting the health and fitness requirements of the National Curriculum for physical education are provided.

Chapter 8 explores the concept of a community and the characteristics of communities that might compromise or promote young people's physical activity. The chapter then turns attention to the potential critical role of the community 'environment' and concludes with an overview of a selection of community-based initiatives or strategies that may enhance young people's physical activity opportunities. Both chapters consider recommendations for promoting physical activity within the school or community context.

Fitness testing is commonplace in both the school and the community setting and has been a topic of much debate in recent years. A number of questions have been raised and concerns expressed over the purpose, value and appropriateness of fitness testing young people. Chapter 9, therefore, considers the key facts, issues and debates on fitness testing, as they relate to encouraging participation in a physically active lifestyle. Given the widespread practice of physical fitness testing in schools in particular, the focus of much of the discussion is on fitness testing within the PE curriculum. To conclude, the chapter provides a series of recommendations on the appropriate use of fitness testing with young people, as well as some alternatives to traditional fitness testing.

The final chapter is divided into two parts. Part one provides an overview and critique of a range of school- and community-based physical activity interventions that have been designed to increase young people's physical activity participation. The outcomes of these initiatives in terms of their impact upon physical, behavioural, cognitive and affective indicators is reviewed, and their trends and characteristics, together with a number of related issues, are highlighted. Finally, in an attempt to assist readers further in the promotion of physical activity in young people, the concluding part of the chapter turns attention to a range of UK initiatives, resources and contact organizations which can support the promotion of physical activity in young people.

Working definitions

The terminology adopted in the area of exercise, health and young people has not always been consistent, and a range of definitions of key terms can be found in the literature. These have been explored to produce the following list of working definitions for the terms that are used throughout this book. Where appropriate, however, some terms are revisited in subsequent chapters in order to debate, clarify and/or extend our understanding of concepts.

Young people

All people aged 5 to 18 years.

Childhood

The period from the first birthday to the onset of puberty.

Adolescence

Adolescence is sometimes used to refer to the psychological changes associated with puberty. Within this text, however, adolescence and puberty are assumed to be synonymous and refer to the period during which a young person experiences the somatic, physical and psychological changes that occur as they develop into adults.

Health

A multifactorial concept which includes dimensions of the physical, mental, social and, some might argue, the spiritual. The World Health Organization has defined health as a state of complete physical, mental and social wellbeing and not merely the absence of disease or infirmity. It is thus seen as a resource for everyday life and as a positive concept emphasizing social and personal resources, as well as physical capacities.

Physical activity

Any bodily movement produced by skeletal muscles that results in energy expenditure. It has dimensions of volume (how much), duration (how long), frequency (how often), intensity (how hard) and mode (what type).

Exercise

A subcomponent of physical activity which is volitional, planned, structured, repetitive and carried out to improve or maintain any aspect of fitness or health.

Sport

A subcomponent of exercise that is rule-governed, structured and competitive, and involves gross motor movement characterized by physical strategy, prowess and chance. In Europe, sport is often used in a wider context to include all exercise and leisure physical activity.

Physical fitness

A set of attributes that people have or achieve that relates to the ability to perform physical activity. Physical fitness has health-related components and performance (skill)-related components. The health-related components of physical fitness include cardiovascular fitness, muscular strength and endurance, flexibility and body composition. The performance-related aspects include agility, balance, co-ordination, power, reaction time and speed. This type of fitness is also sometimes referred to as motor fitness.

Health-related exercise (HRE)

The area of the PE curriculum associated with health and fitness. HRE is physical activity associated with health enhancement and involves the teaching of knowledge, understanding, physical competence and behavioural skills, and the creation of positive attitudes and confidence associated with current and lifelong participation in physical activity.

Health and physical activity promotion

Health promotion incorporates all measures deliberately designed to promote health. It includes health education, plus healthy public policy which aims to achieve social change via legislation, and fiscal, economic and other forms of environmental engineering. Health promotion is concerned with making healthier choices easier choices. In the same vein, and by the same means, physical activity promotion is concerned with making active choices easier choices.

References

HEA (Health Education Authority) (1998) *Young and Active? Policy Framework for Young People and Health-Enhancing Physical Activity.* London: HEA.

Scottish Executive (2003) *Let's Make Scotland More Active. A Strategy for Physical Activity. Physical Activity Task Force.* Edinburgh: The Stationery Office.

2

Young People's Physical Activity and Fitness Status

Lorraine Cale and Jo Harris

There has been considerable interest by researchers, physical educators, health professionals and the media in young people's physical activity and physical fitness in recent years. This is perhaps founded on concerns over young people's activity and fitness status and the possible health consequences. Despite this, and in comparison to adults, there is still relatively little known about young people's activity, fitness and the associated health benefits, and the links between health and physical activity (and physical fitness) which are established in adults, have yet to be confirmed in children (Riddoch, 1998). Indeed, Cavill, Biddle & Sallis (2001) highlight the weaker evidence base for young people and report that there continues to be great debate about the nature and extent of any public health problem. Perhaps as a consequence, a number of myths and misconceptions appear to have developed over the years concerning young people's activity and fitness, often reinforced by the popular media, which, it could be argued, may be misleading the efforts of practitioners and researchers and hindering progress in the field. Nonetheless, the research base on young people is growing (Boreham & Riddoch, 2001). This chapter therefore examines the current evidence surrounding young people's physical activity and physical fitness, and the association between physical activity, physical fitness and health in an attempt to clarify the key findings and issues and dispel any such myths and misconceptions.

Activity

Consider the information and messages that you have acquired to date concerning young people's activity, fitness and health. Read the statements below and establish which you think are true (T) and which you think are false (F). Now study this chapter. As you do so, check your answers with the information presented. Were you as well-informed as you thought?

Statement	T or F?
The onset of cardiovascular disease (CVD) begins in childhood.	
There is overwhelming evidence that physical activity is beneficial to young people's health.	
Physical activity has been found to benefit CVD risk factors, adiposity and bone and psychological health in young people.	
Childhood obesity is neither increasing nor decreasing in most developed countries.	
Some young people are very active whereas others are very inactive.	
Inactive and sedentary lifestyles are common in young people.	
Few young people participate in 30 minutes of moderate physical activity on most days of the week.	
People who are active during their youth are less likely to be active in adulthood.	
There is little evidence that young people today are less active than in previous generations.	
There is little evidence that young people today are less fit than in previous generations.	
Low aerobic fitness is common amongst young people.	
Most boys and girls are not fit enough for health purposes.	

Physical activity, physical fitness and health in young people

The literature on the benefits of physical activity and/or physical fitness to young people's health generally (see Riddoch, 1998; Sallis & Patrick, 1994; Boreham & Riddoch, 2001) and with reference to specific health outcomes (e.g. Alpert & Wilmore, 1994; Armstrong & Simons-Morton, 1994; Mutrie & Parfitt, 1998; Kemper, 2000; Twisk, 2000; Tortolero,

Taylor & Murray, 2000; MacKelvie, Kahn & McKay, 2002) has been reviewed in some detail over the past decade. Blair et al. (1989) proposed a model for the health consequences of childhood physical activity in which three main relationships and benefits arising from adequate physical activity were hypothesized:

1   The direct improvement of childhood health status and quality of life.
2   The direct improvement of adult health status by, for example, delaying the onset of chronic disease in adulthood.
3   An increased likelihood of maintaining adequate activity into adulthood, thus indirectly enhancing adult health status.

The evidence in relation to the first two relationships is reviewed here with respect to various health outcomes. Where data are available, the health consequences of physical fitness are also considered within the model. The latter relationship, commonly referred to as 'tracking', is addressed in the following section of this chapter.

Activity, fitness and current health

Cardiovascular disease (CVD) and risk factors

Studies investigating the relationship between physical activity, physical fitness and cardiovascular health in young people are mostly limited to the study of cardiovascular risk factors as the outcome measure (Twisk, 2000).

Cholesterol and blood pressure   Armstrong & Simons-Morton (1994) reviewed the effects of physical activity on blood lipids in adolescents and concluded that cross-sectional studies indicate a beneficial effect of exercise, but that the results of longitudinal studies are unimpressive. Riddoch (1998) reported physical activity to have only weak associations with serum lipid and lipoprotein concentrations in young people. He revealed six studies which showed no association with measures of activity and six which showed a limited association. More recently, a review by Tolfrey, Jones & Campbell (2000) drew similar conclusions to Armstrong & Simons-Morton (1994). Tolfrey and colleagues (2000) noted that correlational studies suggest that a favourable lipoprotein profile may be related to higher levels of physical activity, but that the majority of longitudinal investigations suggest exercise has little influence. Likewise, Twisk (2000) concluded that there is ambiguous evidence that physical activity and/or physical fitness have some beneficial effects on lipid levels.

In terms of blood pressure, Riddoch (1998) identified seven studies that reported a beneficial association between activity and blood pressure and one that reported no association. Alpert & Wilmore (1994) also analysed the relationship between physical activity and blood pressure, and concluded that aerobic training had only a weak relationship with blood pressure within the normal range. Twisk (2000) suggested there is not much evidence that physical activity and physical fitness have beneficial effects on blood pressure in children and adolescents.

Overweight and obesity   A review of physical activity, adiposity and obesity among adolescents in 1994 concluded that both controlled trials and cross-sectional studies have indicated small but significant beneficial effects of activity for both non-obese and obese adolescents (Bar-Or & Baranowski, 1994). Similarly in a more recent review of the evidence, Riddoch (1998) found that the majority of studies observed some effect. In most, however, beneficial effects were not observed in all assessed parameters and there appeared to be no clear pattern across studies. It was therefore suggested that the results must be treated as highly suggestive rather than definitive (Riddoch, 1998).

In addition, a relationship between cardiovascular fitness and fatness in children has been acknowledged (Twisk, 2000; Boreham & Riddoch, 2001). Boreham & Riddoch (2001) noted a consistently strong relationship between cardiovascular fitness and fatness in studies, and Twisk (2000) concluded from his overview of studies that there is some evidence for a relationship between physical activity, physical fitness and body fatness in children and adolescents.

Bone/skeletal health

Reviews also support the role of physical activity and intervention studies (involving weight-bearing activity) in the promotion of skeletal health and bone mineral density in young people (e.g. Bailey, Faulkner & McKay, 1996; Riddoch, 1998; Bass, 2000; Kemper, 2000; MacKelvie, Kahn & McKay, 2000). Riddoch's review (1998) identified seven studies which showed positive associations between physical activity and parameters related to skeletal health, and three which did not. On the basis of a review of five studies, Kemper (2000) concluded that, whilst research is scarce, recent experimental studies show significant effects of weight-bearing activity and high-impact strength training programmes on site-specific bone mineral density in boys and girls. Similarly, Boreham & Riddoch (2001) suggest that physical activity is an essential stimulus for bone structure, and that it has the potential to increase peak bone mass in children and adolescents. Furthermore, they reported the size of the effect of physical activity (difference in bone mineral density between high and low fitness or activity groups) to be typically between 5 and 15 per cent.

Psychological health

Reviews investigating the link between young people's physical activity (Calfas & Taylor, 1994; Biddle, 1995; Mutrie & Parfitt, 1998), physical fitness (Tortolero, Taylor & Murray, 2000) and psychological health have also been undertaken recently. The review by Calfas & Taylor (1994) found self-esteem, self-concept and depressive symptoms of anxiety/ stress consistently to be related to physical activity. Likewise, the review by Mutrie & Parfitt (1998) reported physical activity to be associated with good mental health (e.g. self-esteem) and low levels of mental health problems (e.g. anxiety, depression) in youth. More recently, Tortolero, Taylor and Murray (2000) reviewed 48 articles and found strong or moderate support for the relationship between activity and fitness in youth in several variables including improved self-efficacy, greater perceived physical competence, greater perceived health and wellbeing, decreases in depression and stress, positive self-concept and positive self-esteem.

Activity, fitness and future health

A few studies have been published recently which have investigated the influence of physical activity and fitness in adolescence on CVD risk factors in later life. For example, the Amsterdam Growth and Health Longitudinal Study (Twisk, Kemper & Van Mechelen, 2002a); the Muscatine Study (Janz, Dawson & Mahoney, 2002); the Northern Ireland Young Hearts Project (Boreham et al., 2002); the Danish Youth and Sports Study (Hasselstrom et al., 2002) and the Leuven Longitudinal Study on Lifestyle, Fitness and Health (Lefevre et al., 2002). The findings suggest that high physical fitness during adolescence and young adulthood is related to a healthy risk factor profile later in life, but that physical activity levels do not influence CVD in later life (Twisk, Kemper & Van Mechelen, 2002b). Thus, although evidence for the influence of fitness on future health appears to be becoming increasingly persuasive, there is no direct proof that activity provides protection from the occurrence of CVD in adulthood (Twisk, 2000; Rowland, 2001).

Boreham & Riddoch (2001), however, suggest that sufficient evidence exists to indicate that childhood physical activity may influence adult disease outcomes in relation to obesity. Following a large-scale study with a 55-year follow-up, Must et al. (1992) reported that overweight in adolescence predicted a wide range of adverse health effects in adulthood that were independent of adult weight. Gunnell et al. (1998) also reported similar findings.

Opinion appears to be mixed as to whether the effects of physical activity on bone density during childhood persist into and benefit adult health. Some consider that the enhanced bone mass from physical activity has the potential to reduce the risk of osteoporosis and associated fractures in later life (Rubin et al., 1993; Boreham & Riddoch, 2001). MacKelvie, Khan & McKay (2002), however, claim that there is currently little research to support this argument.

Finally, evidence linking early physical activity to the development of cancer in adulthood is beginning to emerge. Following a recent review, Culos-Reed (2002) reported that, whilst research is limited and the results did not permit definitive conclusions, participation in regular physical activity during youth appears to have an inverse association with later cancer development.

Summary and considerations

Following his review in 1998, Riddoch (1998, p. 30) concluded that 'no single study, or set of studies, provides definitive evidence for a meaningful health gain through being an active child'. In other words, strong empirical evidence that activity during childhood has a major impact on current or future health has not yet been provided. Evidence is accumulating that more active children generally display healthier cardiovascular profiles, are leaner and develop higher peak bone mass than their less active counterparts (Boreham & Riddoch, 2001), but in many cases the relationships are weak to moderate. In particular, there is little convincing evidence linking childhood activity to adult health. Twisk (2000) concludes that there is weak evidence that physical activity and/or physical fitness are related to a healthy CVD risk profile in children and adolescents. However, he reports that there is no evidence that physical activity and/or physical fitness during childhood and adolescence are related to CVD risk factors in adulthood, or to the occurrence of CVD in adulthood.

Nonetheless, and on a slightly more positive note, Riddoch (1998) suggests that although the inconclusive nature of the evidence may seem disappointing, the associations that do exist are generally in the healthy direction. Furthermore, Boreham & Riddoch (2001) note how evidence is mounting to support the relationships between activity and health and that, in any case, the absence of evidence may not indicate evidence of absence. In other words, subtle relationships may exist which have not been detected.

It is worth considering why the data are not more compelling. Various reasons have been proposed to account for the weak and inconsistent associations with health outcomes. Boreham and Riddoch (2001) suggest that this is largely due to (1) a lack of large-scale longitudinal studies and (2) difficulties in measuring health, fitness and activity in children. The general difficulties in measuring physical activity and physical fitness are discussed in detail in Chapter 3. In addition to these, many studies have assessed the relationship of sustained vigorous activity or exercise training with risk factors but, as this chapter later reveals, young people rarely display this pattern of behaviour (Cavill, Biddle & Sallis, 2001). Also, in the case of young people, health cannot be measured by mortality statistics and epidemiologists are therefore starved of their usual key end points (Fox & Riddoch, 2000). Instead, traditional CVD risk factors are usually relied upon and these are only a relatively crude indicator of coronary health. Most risk factors have a large genetic component (Twisk, 2000) and naturally occurring shifts in CVD risk factors with growth and development can confound relationships (Twisk, 2000; Boreham & Riddoch, 2001). Furthermore, Fox & Riddoch (2000) suggest that for the majority of children it is likely that physical inactivity has not had sufficient time to have had a serious negative influence on risk factors, or that insufficient numbers may be inactive for the effects to be evident. They also note there may be a lack of variability in the health outcomes assessed and where groups are homogenous, statistically significant associations are difficult to identify. In other words, they explain 'you can't make a healthy child healthier' (Fox & Riddoch, 2000, p. 499).

In conclusion though, given the strong and consistent relationships between activity or fitness and health in adults, the paediatric origins of CVD, and the increased prevalence of obesity and other associated conditions in young people in recent years, it would seem likely that adequate physical activity and physical fitness will provide some benefit to young people. Indeed, if one considers the limitations just identified, it could be argued that even small associations may be important.

However, according to Boreham & Riddoch (2001), judgements to date are based largely on limited paediatric data, a richer adult database, educated guesswork and basic physiological principles. Clearly, more substantial research evidence is needed before definitive conclusions can be drawn. Until such a time, we concur with Cavill, Biddle & Sallis (2001 p. 16) who suggest that 'it would be dangerous to conclude that lack of definitive data on the physical health benefits of youth physical activity means that physical activity is not important for their health'. This sentiment might also be echoed for youth physical fitness.

Young people's physical activity

The physical activity levels of young people have been increasingly documented, particularly in the UK, Europe and North America. Despite this, somewhat divergent viewpoints have sometimes developed concerning young people's physical activity. Some consider that today's youth are highly and spontaneously active, that they have endless energy and are constantly on the move (Rowland, 1990; Astrand, 1994), whereas others, perhaps encouraged by media reports, are of the opinion that young people have been habituated into sedentary lifestyles, that their activity levels have declined over the years, and/or that they are not taking sufficient physical activity to benefit their health. That said, it is still generally accepted that activity levels are much higher in young people than in other population groups (Sallis & Owen, 1999). This section endeavours to clarify what is known about young people's physical activity by drawing on the findings and conclusions from a selection of reviews and large-scale international and national studies, as well as some smaller-scale studies. The main findings and consistent trends in the data are highlighted and some key questions concerning young people's physical activity are considered.

Reviews

Cale & Almond (1992a; 1992b; 1992c) conducted a series of reviews on the activity levels of primary, secondary and British children respectively. The conclusions drawn were similar across the reviews. It was noted that young people were not very active and that generally activity levels were low, with many children not taking sufficient exercise to enhance their health status.

Pate, Long & Heath (1994) focused on the physical activity of adolescents and reviewed large population-based studies as well as smaller studies which had used objective monitoring methods (e.g. heart rate). They reported that, on average, adolescents engage in physical activity of any intensity for one hour per day and approximately two thirds of males and a quarter of females participate in moderate to vigorous physical activity for 20 minutes on three or more days per week. Furthermore, they revealed that activity levels decline with increasing age, with the decrease being more marked in females than males. They concluded that, by comparison with adults, adolescents tend to be quite physically active, though age trends indicate that many are at risk of becoming sedentary adults.

Sallis (1993) analysed a selection of self-report studies, including national surveys. He declared males to be 15 to 25 per cent more active than females and activity levels to decrease with age, with the decline to be two and a half times greater in girls than in boys. More recently, Sallis & Owen (1999) provided a further descriptive epidemiology of youth physical activity participation in which the same general trends were noted. They suggested that because physical activity levels are much higher in children and adolescents, very few can be classified as truly sedentary, although many are not sufficiently active to obtain health benefits.

Likewise, Riddoch & Boreham (1995) conducted a review in which virtually all studies reported a decline in activity with age during the teenage years and boys to be more active than girls. However, this latter difference was greatly reduced when moderate activity alone was compared. Further, they suggested that children's activity levels range from very high to very low, with some youngsters being undoubtedly inactive, and others extremely active.

A review by Armstrong & Van Mechelen (1998) also reported similar consistent findings. They noted boys to be more active than girls from an early age and both sexes to reduce their physical activity from childhood through adolescence, with the rate of decline greater in girls. They concluded that some children and adolescents undoubtedly lead sedentary lifestyles but others appear to be active.

More recently, and as part of the European Heart Health Initiative, the European Heart Network commissioned a review of young people and physical activity which included a review of physical activity surveys conducted within the European Union member states (Cavill, 2001). Survey data from Belgium, Denmark, England, Finland, Ireland, the Netherlands, Norway, Sweden and Spain were analysed. In summary,

Cavill (2001) reported that it is clear that many young people are very active and enjoy a great deal of sport and recreation, but that in some countries, especially with boys, polarization of activity is evident, with groups of very active and very inactive adolescents.

Finally, a recent review by Boreham & Riddoch (2001) drew attention to the diverse conclusions that have been reached by researchers following physical activity studies. On the basis of these they claimed 'it is clear that we are currently undecided about (a) how much activity children take; (b) whether children's activity is falling; and (c) whether children's activity is sufficient to promote health' (p. 921). Points (b) and (c) are addressed later in this chapter.

Large-scale international studies

A large multinational WHO study (King & Coles, 1992) involving 11 European countries established the physical activity levels of young people aged 11, 12 and 13 years. The results varied greatly from country to country, and with gender and age. Between approximately 15 and 38 per cent of boys and 20 and 72 per cent of girls were found to exercise less than once a week and a consistent decrease in participation was evident with age, especially among the girls. At all ages studied, fewer girls than boys exercised at least once a week.

Also in 1992, the NHIS–YRBS (US National Health Interview Survey–Youth Risk Behaviour Survey) was conducted on over ten thousand young people aged 12–21 (Department of Health and Human Services & Centers for Disease Control and Prevention, 1996). It revealed that approximately 12 per cent of males and 15 per cent of females had not participated in vigorous or moderate activity during the previous week. The prevalence of inactivity also increased with age. However, approximately 60 per cent of males and 49 per cent of females had participated in vigorous activity on three or more days.

More encouraging findings were reported a few years later in the 1995 school-based US YRBS (Youth Risk Behaviour Survey). The study was again conducted on over ten thousand youngsters, this time aged 15–18. It revealed 7 per cent of males and 14 per cent of females to have engaged in no vigorous or moderate physical activity during the previous week, but 76 per cent and 57 per cent respectively to have participated in vigorous physical activity on at least three days (Department of Health and Human Services & Centers for Disease Control and Prevention, 1996).

In addition, the most recent HBSC (Health Behaviour in School-Aged Children) Study provides comprehensive data on the physical activity patterns of young people (WHO, 2000). This cross-national study involved 26 European countries, plus Canada and the United States, and over a hundred and twenty thousand young people aged 11, 13 and 15. It revealed that about 65 per cent of boys and 47 per cent of girls participated in vigorous exercise two or more times a week and about 80 per cent of boys and 63 per cent of girls participated in vigorous exercise for two or more hours per week. Further, it found that, whilst there was a good deal of variation in physical activity between countries, patterns of involvement, including gender differences, were similar.

Large-scale national studies of young people's physical activity

The Young People and Sport National Survey (2000)

Sport England's most recent National Survey of Young People and Sport was conducted in 1999 (Sport England, 2000), and its findings can be compared to their earlier survey in 1994. In total 3,319 young people aged 6–16 were surveyed. Findings revealed that 79 per cent of young people take part in sport after school, compared with 74 per cent in 1994, and 87 per cent play at least one type of sport 'frequently' (i.e. on ten or more days in the previous year) in their leisure time, the same proportion as in 1994. Furthermore, during the summer holidays just over a quarter of all young people (26 per cent) had taken part in sport and exercise for over 15 hours per week on average (compared with 21 per cent in 1994). The survey also revealed increased participation in extra-curricular sport, from 37 per cent in 1994 to 45 per cent in 1999. Boys' participation was again greater than that of girls.

The Health Survey for England (1997)

The physical activity levels of children (aged 2–15) were assessed within the Health Survey for England for the first time in 1997 (Joint Health Surveys Unit, 1998). The findings revealed that 78 per cent of boys and 70 per cent of girls had participated in some physical activity on five or more days in the previous week. The most common activity type was active play, followed by walking. Overall, boys had spent a mean of 10.41 hours and girls 7.69 hours in physical activities in the previous week. Participation rates among boys and girls declined after about age eight to ten, though the decline was steeper in girls. Participation in vigorous activity (for at least 15 minutes at a time) was reported to be relatively low.

Young People Health-Related Behaviour Survey (2000)

In 2000 the Schools Health Education Unit conducted a large-scale survey on the health-related behaviour, including the physical activity, of 42,073 young people aged between 10 and 15 (Balding, 2001). Over 80 per cent of all young people reported to have exercised and breathed hard at least once in the previous week. The data also revealed that up to 46 per cent of males and up to 33 per cent of females exercised vigorously three times or more a week. Distinct differences between boys' and girls' participation were again evident.

The National Diet and Nutrition Survey (2000)

This nationally representative diet and nutrition survey of 2,127 young people aged 4–18 (Gregory & Lowe, 2000) also gathered physical activity data. The findings revealed girls to be less active than boys and activity levels to decrease with age. On average, boys spent 1.4 hours and girls one hour per day in activities of at least moderate intensity, and 0.4 hours and 0.3 hours per day in vigorous or very vigorous activity respectively. Overall, approximately 40 per cent of boys and 60 per cent of girls spent, on average, less than one hour a day in activities of at least moderate intensity.

What is the nature of young people's physical activity?

The differing nature of young people's physical activity has been recognized in recent years (Rowland, 1998; Welk, Corbin & Dale, 2000). Data from observational studies (e.g. Durant et al., 1993; Bailey et al., 1995) have indicated that young children's activity is highly transitory and that they spend most of their time in low intensity activities interspersed with short bursts of high intensity activity (Armstrong & Welsman, 1997). The study by Bailey et al. (1995), for example, conducted on 6–10-year-olds, revealed that over a hypothetical 12-hour day, children spent most of their time in low intensity activities and an average of 22.3 minutes in high intensity activities. No period of intense activity lasting for ten consecutive minutes was recorded and 95 per cent of intense periods of activity lasted for less than 15 seconds.

Heart rate studies have also confirmed that young people tend to engage primarily in low intensity activity and rarely sustain activity (see Armstrong et al., 1990a; Armstrong & Bray, 1991; Welsman & Armstrong, 1992; McManus & Armstrong, 1995). Within these studies the percentage of time children spent with the heart rate above 139 beats per minute ranged from 4.3 per cent to 9.4 per cent and 38 per cent of boys and 50 per cent of girls did not experience a single sustained ten-minute period with their heart rate above 139 beats per minute over three days (Armstrong & Van Mechelen, 1998).

Has young people's physical activity declined?

As noted earlier, a common assumption and one that has often been reported in the media is that children today are less active than in previous generations. Rowland (2002, p. 1) comments, 'ask anybody on the street, and the answer will probably be the same: Yes, today's youth… are becoming increasingly sedentary and their levels of fitness are in perilous decline.' But, in fact, it is not possible to determine objectively whether young people's physical activity has declined in recent years (Cavill, Biddle & Sallis, 2001). In order to establish this, data must be derived from studies that have employed the same assessment and inter-pretation techniques in similar and representative subject groups, yet such studies are rare (Welsman & Armstrong, 2000). However, one study provides indirect evidence to support this assumption, and data providing further indirect as well as some direct evidence is beginning to emerge. Durnin (1992) pooled energy intake data collected from the 1930s to the 1980s and demonstrated a progressive decrease in the energy intake of adolescents in the UK, but no change in body mass over time. Thus, it is claimed, the only feasible explanation for the marked reduction in energy intake without a change in body mass is that young people's physical activity has decreased over the last 50 years (Armstrong & Van Mechelen, 1998).

Indirect evidence can also be gleaned from analysing changes in young people's lifestyles and travel patterns over time. Young people's freedom to be independently active has decreased in recent years (Hillman, 1993) and fewer children now walk or cycle to school (DiGiuseppi, Roberts & Li 1997; British Heart Foundation, 2000). According to DiGiuseppi, Roberts & Li (1997) such reductions in cycling and walking have undoubtedly contributed to declines in overall physical activity in children.

Research has also emerged recently which has examined changes in activity levels over relatively short periods of time. Welsman & Armstrong (2000) compared young people's physical activity data collected from the same region over ten years apart but found no significant differences in the percentage of time spent in moderate and vigorous activity. They concluded that activity levels do not appear to have fallen dramatically over the past decade. Similarly, the Young People in 2000 Health-Related Behaviour Survey (Balding, 2001) reported fairly consistent results for participation by girls in active sports between 1992 and 2000, and Sport England's National Survey of Young People and Sport (Sport England, 2000) reported participation changes in a positive direction over a five-year period.

Does young people's physical activity influence adult participation?

'Tracking', that is, the notion that physical activity during childhood increases the likelihood of participation as an adult, was identified earlier as one of the proposed benefits arising from childhood physical activity (Blair et al., 1989). Despite this, there is relatively limited evidence available on this issue. Malina (1996) comprehensively reviewed tracking through all stages of the lifespan and concluded that activity tracks weakly to moderately during adolescence, from adolescence into adulthood and across various ages during adulthood. In addition, findings from the Allied Dunbar National Fitness Survey conducted in England (Sports Council & Health Education Authority, 1992) suggest that people who are active in their youth are more likely to be active as adults, while those who are inactive during their youth are unlikely to become physically active adults. The survey revealed that a quarter of those who said they were very active aged 14–19 were currently very active, compared with just two per cent currently active who were inactive at that earlier age. Overall though, the evidence for tracking of activity from childhood is not strong (Boreham & Riddoch, 2001).

Are young people active?

Despite the evidence thus far presented, a key question which still remains is whether young people are 'active' or 'sufficiently active' for health purposes. In this regard, the media have often given the impression that young people are effectively 'couch potatoes'. Whether young people are classified as 'active' or 'inactive' depends on the criteria used (Armstrong & Van Mechelen, 1998), yet, to date, different studies have adopted different criteria in their attempts to answer this question. Based on the population-surveys data they reviewed, Pate, Long & Heath (1994) estimated the extent to which adolescents were meeting the physical activity guidelines for adolescents proposed by Sallis & Patrick (1994) (see Chapter 5 for an overview of physical activity guidelines for young people). They suggested that the vast majority of adolescents meet guideline one (i.e. accumulate 30 minutes of moderate activity on most days) and can be considered reasonably active on a day-to-day basis, but only about 50 per cent meet guideline two (i.e. engage in three or more sessions per week of moderate to vigorous activity for 20 minutes or more at a time).

Armstrong & Van Mechelen (1998) applied the same physical activity guidelines for adolescents to the physical activity data they reviewed. They concluded that most young people satisfy Sallis & Patrick's (1994) recommendation of accumulating 30 minutes of daily moderate intensity activity but few appear regularly to sustain 20-minute periods of activity of moderate to vigorous exertion.

In their review, Riddoch & Boreham (1995) noted how studies using self-report methods indicate that 60–70 per cent of children take sufficient 'appropriate' activity. Overall however, they declared that from the available literature they could not conclude with any degree of certainty whether children are active enough for health purposes.

More recently, the Health Survey for England (Joint Health Surveys Unit, 1998) and the National Diet and Nutrition Survey (Gregory & Lowe, 2000) estimated the percentage of young people meeting the physical activity guidelines for young people proposed by the HEA (i.e. engages in activity of at least moderate intensity for an average of one hour a day) (HEA, 1998). The former study calculated that 55 per cent of boys and 39 per cent of girls achieved recommended levels of physical activity, but that by the age of 15, 29 per cent of boys and 64 per cent of girls were classed as inactive, and the latter reported that approximately 40 per cent of boys and 60 per cent of girls failed to meet the recommendation. Furthermore, in the 15–18 age group, 56 per cent of boys and 69 per cent of girls did not reach the recommendation.

Overall then, this evidence appears to suggest that over half of boys and a third of girls are active and meet current physical activity guidelines, but that still a sizeable number (half and two-thirds, respectively) do not.

Summary and considerations

Evidently, the findings concerning young people's physical activity levels are equivocal, and definitive answers to a number of questions are not available. Reviews and studies have often revealed quite contrasting pictures and drawn different conclusions concerning young people's physical activity. Boreham & Riddoch (2001) ask how it is that such diverse conclusions can be reached by experienced researchers on the basis of well-conducted studies. Explanations they propose include measurement error, different measurement methods, the measurement of different dimensions of physical activity, and population and age-group differences. As Chapter 3 reveals, physical activity is a complex behaviour with different dimensions and there are severe limitations in physical activity measurement techniques, particularly when employed with young people. Thus, the data are limited by the methods available. Indeed, Fox & Riddoch (2000, p. 498) suggest that much of it provides little more than a 'gross estimate' of young people's physical activity.

In addition, the variation in methodology across studies precludes valid, comparative analyses (Armstrong & Welsman, 1997). The studies vary in terms of the nature of the data gathered, the mode of analysis, and the criteria chosen to define 'active', 'inactive' or 'sufficient' activity. On this, Riddoch & Boreham (1995) suggest that analysing the distribution of physical activity levels across a population of children, varying by age and gender, may be more revealing than reported mean or median values of activity obtained from possibly heterogenous groups. Certainly the polarization of activity levels referred to by Cavill (2001) and apparent in a number of the studies reviewed suggests that this may be a more appropriate method of analysis.

The influence the adoption of different criteria can have on young people's reported activity levels has been illustrated in a study by Welk (1994) (cited in Boreham & Riddoch, 2001). Welk (1994) initially reported that only 17 per cent of children achieved a single activity session with a heart rate of above 140 beats per minute. However, when the same results were reanalysed according to health-related criteria, 99 per cent met the criteria. Similarly, Riddoch & Boreham (1995) note the number of different thresholds adopted by studies and how studies using self-report methods indicate higher levels of activity than those using more objective methods.

The variation in methodology and analyses is perhaps not surprising given that the optimal level of physical activity for young people's health has yet to be established (Armstrong & Van Mechelen, 1998) and there is no universal consensus as to what criteria should be adopted (Boreham & Riddoch, 2001). Furthermore, until recently recommendations for the amount of physical activity young people should engage in were not available. Nonetheless, physical activity guidelines for young people have now been developed (see Chapter 5). Also, accompanying these has been a shift of focus from physical activity for the promotion of physical fitness to physical activity for health. This shift however, is not always reflected in the physical activity data reported. Indeed, it could be argued that the data that have been collected and reported in some studies are not the most useful, meaningful or relevant, and fail to allow clear conclusions to be drawn concerning young people's physical activity. It would be helpful to practitioners if some consensus could be established amongst researchers with respect to the nature of activity information that should be gathered and the criteria that should be applied to denote 'active'/'inactive'. Until further evidence becomes available, the current physical activity guidelines for young people (see Chapter 5) would seem to be the most appropriate criteria to adopt. Not surprisingly, a few of the larger-scale surveys (e.g. Joint Health Surveys Unit, 1998; Gregory & Lowe, 2000) have adopted these.

The above limitations aside, however, it is possible to identify key findings and a number of consistent trends within the literature. These are summarized in Table 2.1.

Table 2.1   A summary of the key findings and trends concerning young people and physical activity

Over half of boys and over a third of girls appear to be active and meet current physical activity guidelines for young people, but a sizeable proportion (half of boys and two-thirds of girls) are inactive and lead sedentary lifestyles.
National and international surveys reveal relatively good levels of participation in a number of young people.
Polarization of activity in young people appears to be common, with groups of very active and very inactive youngsters.
Boys are more active than girls.
Physical activity declines with age – the teenage years appear to be the ages of greatest decline.
Young people's activity patterns appear to be sporadic and highly transitory – most of their time is spent in low intensity activity and they seldom experience sustained periods of moderate to vigorous activity.
It cannot be firmly established whether young people's physical activity has declined over previous generations or whether it has declined over recent years.
The evidence for tracking of activity from childhood is not strong – activity tracks weakly to moderately during adolescence, and from adolescence into adulthood.

Discussion point   Consider the key findings shown in Table 2.1. Are you surprised by any? If so, which?

On the basis of the findings:

1   Do you feel the promotion of physical activity in young people is warranted/justified?
2   What do you feel the priorities of physical educators, health professionals and others working with young people should be?

Explain your reasons.

It is interesting to note that a number of studies show good participation levels (e.g. Department of Health and Human Services & Centers for Disease Control and Prevention, 1996; Sport England, 2000; WHO, 2000) and many young people to be meeting current physical activity guidelines (e.g. Pate, Long & Health, 1994; Joint Health Surveys Unit, 1998; Gregory & Lowe, 2000). However, whilst these results may seem encouraging on the surface, still a sizeable proportion of young people within these and other studies are inactive and lead sedentary lifestyles. For example, the Health Survey for England revealed that by the age of 15, 29 per cent of boys and 64 per cent of girls were classed as inactive (Joint Health Surveys Unit, 1998) and in the National Diet and Nutrition Survey (Gregory & Lowe, 2000) 56 per cent of boys and 69 per cent of girls aged 15–18 did not achieve the recommended level of activity. In this respect, and as was acknowledged by Cavill (2001), it is a concern to see an apparent polarization of activity in young people, with some undoubtedly very active youngsters and some very inactive.

Clear trends are evident from the data for both gender and age, and these are consistent across studies. Boys are more active than girls and activity declines with age. According to Sallis (2000), the age-related decline in physical activity may be the most consistent finding in physical activity epidemiology. More recently however, the commonly reported finding that the decline is more marked in girls than boys has been refuted (Sallis, 2000). A symposium focusing on four papers confirmed the near universality of the decline in activity and identified the teen years (13–18) as the period of greatest decline, but concluded that the decline was generally greater for males than females and greater in vigorous activities and in non-organized sports activities (Sallis, 2000).

Finally, another commonly accepted finding is that young people are intermittently active, that their activity patterns are sporadic, and that they seldom experience sustained periods of moderate to vigorous activity

(Armstrong & Van Mechelen, 1998). However, currently much of this evidence comes from objective studies conducted on young children, often with limited sample sizes. It would be useful to know *when* the nature of young people's physical activity begins to change to reflect adult patterns.

Young people's physical fitness

Physical fitness comprises health-related and performance (skill)-related components (Caspersen, Powell & Christenson, 1985) which, as is explained in Chapter 3, can be measured via laboratory or field tests. The health-related components, and more specifically aerobic fitness, are of interest here because they are related to specific 'health' or disease outcomes (Pate, 1988). Also, given that field measures are not considered suitable for the assessment of single, basic, physiological functions (Astrand & Rodahl, 1987), the studies reviewed are restricted to those which focus on laboratory measures of aerobic fitness. Peak oxygen uptake (peak VO_2), the highest rate at which an individual can consume oxygen during exercise, limits the capacity to perform aerobic exercise and is widely recognized as the best single measure of young people's aerobic fitness (Armstrong & Welsman, 1994).

The measurement of young people's aerobic fitness has been afforded a good deal of attention over the years, with the first laboratory-based studies being conducted between 50 and 65 years ago (Robinson, 1938; Morse, Schlutz & Cassels, 1949; Astrand, 1952). These have since been supplemented by a number of cross-sectional studies as well as several longitudinal studies from most parts of the world (Armstrong & Welsman, 1997; Armstrong & Van Mechelen, 1998). A number of recent reviews have summarized the data available (e.g. Rowland, 1993; Armstrong & Welsman, 1994; Welsman & Armstrong, 1996; Armstrong & Welsman, 1997; Armstrong & Van Mechelen, 1998; Armstrong & Welsman, 2000a; 2000b).

Aerobic fitness and age

The review by Armstrong & Welsman (1994) examined data from the literature collected during the period 1938–93 and generated graphs representing well over four thousand treadmill-determined peak VO_2 scores of untrained 8–16-year-olds in relation to age. Data from both cross-sectional and longitudinal studies with varying sample sizes were included which revealed an almost linear increase in peak VO_2 with age in both boys and girls. According to Armstrong & Welsman (2000a), however, several cross-sectional studies have indicated a decline or at least a levelling-off in girls' peak VO_2 between the ages of 13 and 15.

Few substantial longitudinal studies of young people's peak VO_2 have been carried out, but the data are in general agreement with the cross-sectional studies (Armstrong & Welsman 2000b). They again provide a consistent picture of a progressive rise in boys' peak VO_2 with age. For example, Mirwald & Bailey (1986) reported an average annual increase in peak VO_2 of 11 per cent in boys, whilst Armstrong & Welsman (1994) noted a 36 per cent increase in peak VO_2 in boys between 11 and 13 years. Within the former study, girls demonstrated a similar trend from 8 to 13 years, and averaged an annual increase in peak VO_2 of 12 per cent. However, longitudinal studies with older girls have also shown a levelling-off or even a decline in girls' peak VO_2 from about 14 years (Armstrong & Welsman, 2000a).

Aerobic fitness and growth and maturation

Peak VO_2 is highly related to body size and conventionally studies have attempted to control for differences in body size by simply expressing peak VO_2 in relation to mass as millilitres of oxygen per kilogram body mass per minute (i.e. ml kg^{-1} min^{-1}). Data from such studies are consistent and demonstrate that between the ages of 8 and 18, boys' mass-related peak VO_2 remains unchanged at approximately 50 ml kg^{-1} min^{-1} whereas girls' values experience a progressive decline from about 45 to 35 ml kg^{-1} min^{-1} (Armstrong & Welsman, 2000a).

The validity of simple ratio scaling to remove the influence of body mass effects has been questioned however, and studies in which the influence of body size has been removed using appropriate allometric techniques may provide a clearer, more accurate picture of growth-related peak VO_2 (Armstrong & Welsman, 2000a). Welsman et al. (1996) used both traditional ratio and allometric scaling to remove the effects of body size from peak VO_2 in groups of prepubertal and circumpubertal boys and girls and adults. The results of the traditional analyses conformed with the findings above, but a different picture emerged from the allometric analyses. Peak VO_2 significantly increased into puberty with no decline into adulthood.

More recently, the emergence of multilevel modelling techniques has enabled body size, age and sex effects to be portioned concurrently within an allometric framework in order better to understand longitudinal data (Armstrong & Welsman, 2000b). Armstrong et al. (1999) applied multilevel modelling to the interpretation of peak VO_2 in 11–13-year-olds. In accordance with the cross-sectional findings of Welsman et al. (1996), the data demonstrated a progressive increase in aerobic fitness in boys and girls over the age range, independent of the influence of body size.

Relatively few studies have investigated the relationship between peak VO_2 and maturation (Armstrong & Welsman, 2000b) and data derived using appropriate scaling techniques to partition body size effects are limited (Armstrong & Welsman, 2000a). Armstrong, Welsman & Kirby (1998) determined the peak VO_2 of 93 male and 83 female 12-year-olds. In accordance with the extant literature, the authors found that peak VO_2 in ratio with body mass remained unchanged with maturation. However, when body mass was accounted for using allometry, peak VO_2 significantly increased with maturation in boys and girls and indicated an additional effect of maturation on peak VO_2, above that due to growth.

Armstrong and colleagues have also recently introduced stage of maturation into a multilevel regression model of 11–13 and 11–17-year-olds' peak VO_2 respectively (Armstrong et al., 1999; Armstrong & Welsman, 2001). Again, with body size and fatness allowed for, peak VO_2 increased with age and maturation in both sexes. Thus, although this data is limited and conflicts with the traditional interpretation, Armstrong & Welsman (2000a) suggest that the results provide convincing and consistent evidence that relative to body size, peak aerobic fitness increases progressively in boys throughout childhood and adolescence into adulthood, and in girls increases at least into puberty, and that the maturational process itself induces increases in aerobic fitness over and above those explained by size, body fatness and age.

Aerobic fitness and sex

The evidence that boys have a higher peak VO_2 than girls, regardless of how it is examined and expressed, is compelling (Armstrong & Welsman, 2000b). If boys' and girls' peak VO_2 data is compared at various ages, boys' values are about 12 per cent higher than girls' at ten years, with the sex difference becoming more pronounced during the teen years, typically reaching 37 per cent at 16 years of age (Armstrong & Welsman, 2000b). Longitudinal studies also support this trend. With the influence of body size appropriately removed, boys' peak VO_2 increases from prepuberty, through puberty and into the early adult years, whereas girls' peak VO_2 increases from prepuberty into circumpuberty but then levels off (Welsman et al., 1996).

Are young people fit?

That young people are 'unfit' and/or their aerobic fitness has declined over the years has perhaps been even more widely documented in the media than the common (yet unfounded) claims concerning young people's physical activity. Also, as with physical activity, there is no consensus on the optimal level of physical fitness for young people. However, experts drawn from the European Pediatric Work Physiology Group suggested that it may be possible to express a lower limit of peak VO_2 that, in the absence of other health-related problems, may represent a 'health risk' (Bell et al., 1986). Risk levels of 35 ml kg^{-1} min^{-1} and 30 ml kg^{-1} min^{-1} were proposed for boys and girls respectively. Regrettably, few studies have reported results in sufficient detail to determine the percentage of young people falling below these thresholds. Nonetheless, some estimates have been made. For example, a reanalysis of data collected over a ten-year period on over two and a half thousand young people in relation to these 'health-risk' thresholds revealed that only about 2 per cent of young people aged 9 to 16 could be classified as at risk (Armstrong et al., 1990b; Armstrong et al., 1991; Armstrong et al., 1996), and another study of prepubertal children reported that all had values above the 'health-risk' threshold (Armstrong et al., 1995). Furthermore, in analysing the mean values obtained in longitudinal studies of aerobic fitness, it is evident that all comfortably exceed the health-risk threshold values proposed by Bell et al. (1986) (see Armstrong & Van Mechelen, 1998). Thus, there appears to be no evidence to suggest that low levels of aerobic fitness are common amongst young people.

Has young people's fitness declined?

According to Rowland (2002), the concept that physical fitness (and physical activity) have been decreasing in youth over the last half century is not limited to public perception but has been supported by professional opinion as well. He questions, however, whether the decline in aerobic fitness is fact or supposition. Regrettably, despite a few researchers addressing this question in recent years (e.g. Armstrong & Welsman,

1997; Armstrong & Van Mechelen, 1998; Rowland, 2002), the research is disappointingly scant (Rowland, 2002).

Based on an analysis of data over almost six decades, Armstrong & Welsman (1997) and Armstrong & Van Mechelen (1998) report that there is no scientific evidence to suggest that young people's aerobic fitness has declined over the last 50 years. They noted how the aerobic fitness of young people appears to have remained remarkably consistent over time, with the current data closely reflecting the findings of earlier studies.

Likewise, following his review of the evidence, Rowland (2002) concluded that the existing research literature does not permit any confident conclusions to be drawn regarding temporal changes in aerobic fitness. He reviewed changes in aerobic fitness in youth, as defined by both endurance performance and maximal aerobic power. He suggested that studies of changes in endurance performance, as measured via fitness test batteries, have provided conflicting and not particularly convincing findings. His summary of aerobic power data from a number of studies of boys over a 30-year period confirmed the findings of Armstrong & Welsman (1997) and Armstrong & Van Mechelen (1998). No obvious changes in either direction were evident and the values were remarkably similar to the earliest values reported by Robinson (1938). As a result, he declared that there is no evidence that VO_2 max values in children have changed over the years.

Summary and considerations

As with physical activity, the assessment and interpretation of young people's physical fitness, as determined via aerobic fitness, is complex and has limitations (see Chapter 3, Table 3.1). Aside from the difficulties however, Armstrong & Welsman (2000b) suggest that peak VO_2 can be accepted as a maximal index of aerobic fitness in older children or adolescents provided certain procedures are followed. Nonetheless, the data should be interpreted cautiously. No information is available on randomly selected groups of young people, and since volunteers are generally used as subjects in studies, selection bias cannot be ruled out (Armstrong & Welsman, 2000a). Rowland (2002) likewise acknowledges the limitations with data that is not population-representative. In analysing temporal changes in aerobic fitness, he also cautions the methodology of comparing data over time from different laboratories with different equipment, protocols and staff. Given the limitations, he claims, trying to detect small changes in fitness 'would seem almost impossible' (Rowland, 2002, p. 6).

A further issue relates to the influence in particular of heredity or genetic potential and maturation on young people's aerobic fitness (see Chapter 3 for a more detailed overview of the influence of these and other factors on physical fitness). Indeed, and again with respect to changes in aerobic fitness over time, Blair (1995) suggested that it is unlikely that significant population changes would occur in such genetically determined performance characteristics. Similarly, because extra adipose tissue serves as a load which must be transported during weight-bearing activity, increases in body weight and body fatness associated with maturation will have a negative influence on tests of aerobic capacity (Rowland, 2002) if, as highlighted earlier, they are not accounted for.

Whilst recognizing the limitations, it is still possible and important to highlight some of the key findings from the literature. Based on the evidence to date and the reviews and summaries of various authors (e.g. Armstrong & Welsman, 1997; 2000a; 2000b; Rowland, 2002), Table 2.2 summarizes the key findings concerning young people's aerobic fitness.

Table 2.2   A summary of the key findings concerning young people and aerobic fitness

Young people show a progressive, almost linear increase in peak VO_2 with age, although some studies show that from about 14 years, girls' peak VO_2 levels off or declines.
With body size appropriately controlled for, boys' peak VO_2 increases through childhood and adolescence and into early adulthood, whilst that of girls increases into puberty and then levels off.
Whilst data are limited, evidence indicates that maturation induces increases in peak VO_2 in both sexes, independent of those explained by body size, body fatness and age.
Boys' peak VO_2 is higher than that of girls at least from late childhood, and there is a progressive divergence in boys' and girls' values during the teenage years.
There is no evidence to suggest that low levels of aerobic fitness are common amongst young people.
There is no convincing evidence to suggest that young people's aerobic fitness has declined over time.

Discussion point   Consider the key findings shown in Table 2.2. Address the same questions as earlier (see previous discussion point on p. 26), but for physical fitness and young people.

Physical fitness or physical activity?

A final debate concerns whether there is a need to focus on the promotion of physical activity or physical fitness in young people, or indeed both. Arguably, media messages to date have tended to favour the notion of 'getting young people fitter'. Given the evidence presented here though, where should physical educators, and health and other professionals be directing their energies and efforts?

More recently and for various reasons, a number of researchers have advocated the promotion of physical activity rather than physical fitness. For example, given that there is no evidence that low levels of aerobic fitness are common amongst young people or that fitness has declined over the past 50 years, Cavill, Biddle & Sallis (2001) suggest that, for public health purposes, it is more important to monitor young people's participation in physical activity than to monitor fitness. Indeed, this view is also supported by the evidence from studies of young people's physical activity which has revealed many young people to be inactive and a sizeable proportion to be failing to meet current physical activity recommendations. Riddoch & Boreham (1995), meanwhile, suggest that physical activity rather than physical fitness is the most important variable to assess because of the contributions to fitness of genetic influences, maturational status, and activity levels.

Others have cited sound behavioural reasons for focusing on physical activity rather than fitness (e.g. Rowland, 1995; Pangrazi, 2000; Cale & Harris, 2002; Corbin, 2002). These are explored in detail in Chapter 9 but suffice it to say that emphasizing fitness may be counterproductive to the promotion of active lifestyles in young people and have as many negative consequences as positive ones (Rowland, 1990; Corbin, 2002). Such a focus has also been unsuccessful in the past (Pangrazi, 2000). In contrast to physical fitness (an attribute), increased physical activity (a behaviour) is an outcome that can be accomplished by all young people (Pangrazi, 2000) and is therefore more likely to be acceptable to the general public, particularly to the sedentary or less fit (Rowland, 1995).

Another factor relevant to this debate is whether one is more important to health than the other, i.e. is fitness or activity more important to health? According to Boreham & Riddoch (2001), the question of whether physical activity or physical fitness is more strongly related to health status remains unresolved. Nonetheless, the evidence that fitness is related to health itself, without being mediated by physical activity, is becoming increasingly persuasive and high cardiorespiratory fitness may be directly related to improved health status (Boreham & Riddoch, 2001). As acknowledged earlier, recent findings suggest that high physical fitness during adolescence and young adulthood is related to a healthy CVD risk profile in later life, but that physical activity levels do not influence CVD risk in later life (Twisk, Kemper & Van Mechelen, 2002b). This could lead some to conclude that, from the point of view of future health, it may be better to focus on physical fitness rather than physical activity in youth. However, this association may in part be genetically determined and be independent of activity. For instance, a high-fit individual could automatically be blessed with better health status and conversely a low-fit individual could be unfortunate enough to have poorer health. According to Boreham & Riddoch (2001), an alternative, but not mutually exclusive, explanation might be that fitness acts as a marker for high activity, which might not only improve cardiovascular function but also promote changes in other health indicators (e.g. lower blood pressure).

In summary, both physical activity and physical fitness are clearly desirable for young people, and trying to promote and ensure adequate amounts of both should be beneficial, if approached in an appropriate way. However, given the evidence and issues outlined, plus the reality of the limited time and resources often available to physical educators, and health and other practitioners working with young people, in our view, and as a priority, more attention and energy should be devoted to 'getting more young people active or more active', than to 'getting them fitter'!

References

Alpert, B. S. & Wilmore, J. H. (1994) Physical activity and blood pressure in adolescents, *Pediatric Exercise Science*, **6**, 361–80.

Armstrong, N., Balding, J., Gentle, P. & Kirby, B. (1990a) Patterns of Physical activity among 11 to 16 year old British children, *British Medical Journal*, **301**, 203–5.

Armstrong, N., Balding, J., Gentle, P. & Kirby, B. (1990b) Estimation of coronary risk factors in British school children: a preliminary report, *British Journal of Sports Medicine*, **24**, 61–6.

Armstrong, N. & Bray, S. (1991) Physical activity patterns defined by continuous heart rate monitoring, *Archives of Disease in Childhood*, **66**, 245–7.

Armstrong, N., Kirby, B. J., McManus, A. M. & Welsman, J. R. (1995) Aerobic fitness of pre-pubescent children, *Annals of Human Biology*, **22**, 427–41.

Armstrong, N., Kirby, B., McManus, A. & Welsman, J. (1996) Physical activity patterns and aerobic fitness among pre-pubescents, *European Physical Education Review*, **7**, 19–29.

Armstrong, N. & Simons-Morton, B. (1994) Physical activity and blood lipids in adolescents, *Pediatric Exercise Science*, **6**, 381–405.

Armstrong, N. & Van Mechelen, W. (1998) Are young people fit and active? In Biddle, S., Sallis, J. & Cavill, N. (eds), *Young and Active? Young People and Health-Enhancing Physical Activity – Evidence and Implications*. London: Health Education Authority, 69–97.

Armstrong, N. & Welsman, J. R. (1994) Assessment and interpretation of aerobic fitness in children and adolescents, *Exercise and Sports Sciences Reviews*, **22**, 435–76.

Armstrong, N. & Welsman, J. (1997) *Young People and Physical Activity*. Oxford: Oxford University Press.

Armstrong, N. & Welsman, J. R. (2000a) Aerobic Fitness. In Armstrong, N. & Van Mechelen, W. (eds), *Paediatric Exercise Science and Medicine*. Oxford: Oxford University Press, 173–82.

Armstrong, N. & Welsman, J. R. (2000b) Development of aerobic fitness during childhood and adolescence, *Pediatric Exercise Science*, **12**, 128–49.

Armstrong, N. & Welsman, J. R. (2001) Peak oxygen uptake in relation to growth and maturation in 11- to 17-year-old humans, *European Journal of Applied Physiology*, **85**, 546–51.

Armstrong, N., Welsman, J. R. & Kirby, B. J. (1998) Peak oxygen uptake and maturation in 12 year olds, *Medicine and Science in Sports and Exercise*, **30**, 165–9.

Armstrong, N., Welsman, J. R., Nevill, A. M. & Kirby, B. J. (1999) Modeling growth and maturation changes in peak oxygen uptake in 11–13 year olds, *Journal of Applied Physiology*, **87**, 2230–6.

Armstrong, N., Williams, J., Balding, J., Gentle, P. & Kirby, B. (1991) The peak oxygen uptake of British children with reference to age, sex, and sexual maturity, *European Journal of Applied Physiology*, **62**, 369–75.

Astrand, P. O. (1952) *Experimental Studies of Physical Working Capacity in Relation to Sex and Age*. Copenhagen: Munksgaard.

Astrand, P. O. (1994) Physical activity and fitness: evolutionary perspective and trends for the future. In Bouchard, C., Shephard, R. J. & Stephens, T. (eds), *Physical Activity, Fitness, and Health: International Proceedings and Consensus Statement*. Champaign, IL: Human Kinetics, pp. 98–105.

Astrand, P. O. & Rodahl, K. (1987) *Textbook of Work Physiology*. New York: McGraw Hill.

Bailey, D. A., Faulkner, R. A. & McKay, H. A. (1996) Growth, physical activity and bone mineral acquisition, *Exercise and Sports Science Reviews*, **24**, 233–66.

Bailey, R. C., Olson, J., Pepper, S. L., Porszaz, J., Barstow, T. L. & Cooper, D. M. (1995) The level and tempo of children's physical activities: an observation study, *Medicine and Science in Sports and Exercise*, **27**,1033–41.

Balding, J. (2001) *Young People in 2000*. Exeter: Schools Health Education Unit.

Bar-Or, O. & Baranowski, T. (1994) Physical activity, adiposity and obesity among adolescents, *Pediatric Exercise Science*, **6**, 348–60.

Bass, S. L. (2000) The prepubertal years. A uniquely opportune stage of growth when the skeleton is most responsive to exercise? *Sports Medicine*, **30(2)**, 73–8.

Bell, R. D., Macek, M., Rutenfranz, J. & Saris, W. H. M. (1986) Health indicators and risk factors of cardiovascular diseases during childhood and adolescence. In Rutenfranz, J., Mocellin, R. & Klimt, F. (eds), *Children and Exercise XII*, Champaign, IL: Human Kinetics, 19–27.

Biddle, S. (1995) Exercise and psychosocial health, *Research Quarterly for Exercise and Sport*, **66**, 292–7.

Blair, S. N. (1995) Youth fitness: directions for future research. In Cheung, L. W. Y. & Richmond, J. B. (eds), *Child Health, Nutrition and Physical Activity*. Champaign, IL: Human Kinetics, 147–52.

Blair, S. N., Clark, D. G., Cureton, K. J. & Powell, K. E. (1989) Exercise and fitness in childhood: implications for a lifetime of health. In Gisolfi, C. V., & Lamb, D. R. (eds), *Perspectives in Exercise Science and Sports Medicine, Vol. 2: Youth, Exercise and Sport*. New York: McGraw-Hill.

Boreham, C. & Riddoch, C. (2001) The physical activity, fitness and health of children, *Journal of Sports Sciences*, **19**, 915–29.

Boreham, C., Twisk, J., Neville, C., Savage, M., Murray, L. & Gallagher, A. (2002) Associations between physical fitness and activity patterns during adolescence and cardiovascular risk factors in young adulthood: The Northern Ireland Young Hearts Project, *International Journal of Sports Medicine*, **23**(supplement), S22–6.

British Heart Foundation. (2000) Couch Kids. *The Growing Epidemic: Looking at Physical Activity in Children in the UK*. London: The British Heart Foundation.

Cale, L. & Almond, L. (1992a) Physical activity levels of young children: a review of the evidence, *Health Education Journal*, **51(2)**, 94–9.

Cale, L. & Almond, L. (1992b) Physical activity levels of secondary-aged children: a review, *Health Education Journal*, **51(4)**, 192–7.

Cale, L. & Almond, L. (1992c) Children's activity levels: a review conducted on British children, *Physical Education Review*, **15(2)**, 111–18.

Cale, L. & Harris, J. (2002) National fitness testing for children – issues, concerns and alternatives, *The British Journal of Teaching Physical Education*, **33(1)**, 32–4.

Calfas, K. J. & Taylor, C. (1994) Effects of physical activity on psychological variables in adolescents, *Pediatric Exercise Science*, **6**, 406–23.

Caspersen, C. J., Powell, K. E. & Christenson, G. M. (1985) Physical activity, exercise and physical fitness: definitions and distinctions for health-related research, *Public Health Reports*, **100**, 126–30.

Cavill, N. (2001) Children and Young People – The Importance of Physical Activity. A paper published in the context of the European Heart Health Initiative. Brussels: European Heart Network.

Cavill, N., Biddle, S. & Sallis, J. F. (2001) Health enhancing physical activity for young people: statement of the United Kingdom Expert Consensus Conference, *Pediatric Exercise Science*, **13**, 12–25.

Corbin, C. B. (2002) Physical activity for everyone: what every physical educator should know about promoting lifelong physical activity, *Journal of Teaching in Physical Education*, **21**, 128–44.

Culos-Reed, S. N. (2002) Physical activity and cancer in youth: a review of physical activity's protective and rehabilitative functions, *Pediatric Exercise Science*, **14**, 248–58.

Department of Health and Human Services & Centers for Disease Control and Prevention (1996) *Physical Activity and Health: A Report of the Surgeon General.* Atlanta, GA:.

DiGuiseppi, C., Roberts, I. & Li, L. (1997) Influence of changing travel patterns on child death rates from injury: trend analysis, *British Medical Journal*, **314**, 710–13.

Durant, R. H., Baranowski, T., Rohdes, T., Gutin, B., Thompson, W. O., Carroll, R., Puhl, J. & Greaves, K. A. (1993) Association among serum lipid and lipoprotein concentrations and physical activity. Physical fitness and body composition in young children, *Journal of Pediatrics*, **123**, 185–92.

Durnin, J. V. G. A. (1992) Physical activity levels past and present. In Norgan, N. (ed.), *Physical Activity and Health*. Cambridge: Cambridge University Press, 20–7.

Fox, K. R. & Riddoch, C. (2000) Charting the physical activity patterns of contemporary children and adolescents, *Proceedings of the Nutrition Society*, **59**, 497–504.

Gregory, J. & Lowe, S. (2000) *National Diet and Nutrition Survey: Young People Aged 4 to 18 Years*. London: The Stationery Office.

Gunnell, D. J., Frankel, S. J., Nanchahal, K., Peters, T. J. & Davey-Smith, G. (1998) Childhood obesity and adult cardiovascular mortality: a 57-y follow-up study based on the Boyd-Orr cohort, *American Journal of Clinical Nutrition*, **67**, 1111–18.

Hasselstrom, H., Hansen, S. E., Froberg, K. & Andersen, L. B. (2002) Physical fitness and physical activity during adolescence as predictors of cardiovascular disease risk in young adulthood: Danish Youth Sports Study: An eight-year follow-up study, *International Journal of Sports Medicine*, **23**(supplement), S27–31.

HEA (Health Education Authority) (1998) *Young and Active? Policy Framework for Young People and Health-Enhancing Physical Activity*. London: HEA.

Hillman, M. (1993) One false move...An overview of the findings and issues they raise. In *Children, Transport and the Quality of Life*. London: Policy Studies Institute, 7–18.

Janz, K. F., Dawson, J. D. & Mahoney, L. T. (2002) Increases in physical fitness during childhood improves cardiovascular health during adolescence: The Muscatine Study, *International Journal of Sports Medicine*, **23** (supplement), S15–21.

Joint Health Surveys Unit (1998) *Health Survey for England: The Health of Young People 1995–1997*. London: HMSO.

Kemper, H. C. G. (2000) Physical activity and bone health. In Armstrong, N. & Van Mechelen, W. (eds), *Paediatric Exercise Science and Medicine*. Oxford: Oxford University Press, 265–72.

King, A. J. C. & Coles, B. (1992) *The Health of Canada's Youth*. Canada: Ministry of Health and Welfare.

Lefevre, J., Philippaerts, R., Delvaux, K., Thomis, M., Claessens, A. L., Lysens, R. et al. (2002) Relation between cardiovascular risk factors at adult age, and physical activity during youth and adulthood. The Leuven Longitudinal Study on Lifestyle, Fitness and Health. *International Journal of Sports Medicine*, **23**(supplement), S32–8.

MacKelvie, K. J., Kahn, K. M. & McKay, H. A. (2002) Is there a critical period for bone response to weight-bearing exercise in children and adolescents? A systematic review, *British Journal of Sports Medicine*, **36**, 250–7.

Malina, R. M. (1996) Tracking of physical activity and physical fitness across the lifespan, *Research Quarterly for Exercise and Sport*, **67**(supplement), S1–10.

McManus, A. & Armstrong, N. (1995) Patterns of physical activity among primary schoolchildren. In Ring, F. J. (ed.), *Children in Sport*. Bath: Bath University Press, 17–23.

Mirwald, R. L. & Bailey, D. A. (1986) *Maximal Aerobic Power*. London and Ontario: Sports Dynamics.

Morse, M., Schlutz, F. W. & Cassels, D. E. (1949) Relation of age to physiological responses of the older boy to exercise, *Journal of Applied Physiology*, **1**, 683–709.

Must, A., Jacques, P. F., Dallal, G. E., Bajema, C. J. & Dietz, W. H. (1992) Long-term mobidity and mortality of overweight adolescents, *New England Journal of Medicine*, **327**, 1350–5.

Mutrie, N. & Parfitt, G. (1998) Physical activity and its link with mental, social and moral health in young people. In Biddle, S., Sallis, J. & Cavill, N. (eds), *Young and Active? Young People and Health-Enhancing Physical Activity – Evidence and Implications*. London: Health Education Authority, 49–68.

Pangrazi, R. P. (2000) Promoting physical activity for youth, *The ACHPER Healthy Lifestyles Journal*, **47**(2), 18–21.

Pate, R. R. (1988) The evolving definition of physical fitness, *Quest*, **40**, 174–9.

Pate, R. R., Long, B. J., & Heath, G. (1994) Descriptive epidemiology of physical activity in adolescents, *Pediatric Exercise Science*, **6**, 434–47.

Riddoch, C. (1998) Relationships between physical activity and physical health in young people. In Biddle, S., Sallis, J. & Cavill, N. (eds), *Young and Active? Young People and Health-Enhancing Physical Activity – Evidence and Implications.* London: Health Education Authority, 17–48.

Riddoch, C. & Boreham, C. A. G. (1995) The health-related physical activity of children, *Sports Medicine*, **19(2)**, 86–102.

Robinson, S. (1938) Experimental studies of physical fitness in relation to age, *Arbeitsphysiologie*, **10**, 251–323.

Rowland, T. W. (1990) *Exercise and Children's Health.* Champaign, IL: Human Kinetics.

Rowland, T. W. (1993) Aerobic exercise testing protocols. In Rowland, T. W. (ed.), *Pediatric Laboratory Exercise Testing*, Champaign, IL: Human Kinetics, 19–41.

Rowland, T. W. (1995) The horse is dead; let's dismount, *Pediatric Exercise Science*, **7**, 117–20.

Rowland, T. W. (1998) The biological basis of physical activity, *Medicine and Science in Sports and Exercise*, **30**, 392–9.

Rowland, T. W. (2001) The role of physical activity and fitness in children in the prevention of adult cardiovascular disease, *Progress in Pediatric Cardiology*, **12**, 199–203.

Rowland, T. W. (2002) Declining cardiorespiratory fitness in youth: fact or supposition? *Pediatric Exercise Science*, **14**, 1–8.

Rubin, K., Schirduan, V., Gendreau, P., Sarfarazi, M., Medola, R. & Dalksy, G. (1993) Predictors of axial and peripheral bone mineral density in healthy children and adolescents, with special attention to the role of puberty, *Journal of Pediatrics*, **123**, 863–70.

Sallis, J. F. (1993) Epidemiology of physical activity and fitness in children and adolescents, *Critical Reviews in Food Science and Nutrition*, **33**, 403–8.

Sallis, J. F. (2000) Age-related decline in physical activity: a synthesis of human and animal studies, *Medicine and Science in Sports and Exercise*, **32**, 1598–1600.

Sallis, J. F. & Owen, N. (1999) The descriptive epidemiology of physical activity participation by youth. In Sallis, J. F. & Owen, N. (eds), *Physical Activity and Behavioural Medicine.* Thousand Oaks: Sage, 102–6.

Sallis, J. F. & Patrick, K. (1994) Physical activity guidelines for adolescents: consensus statement, *Pediatric Exercise Science*, **6**, 302–14.

Sport England (2000) *Young People and Sport. National Survey 1999.* London: Sport England.

Sports Council & Health Education Authority (1992) *Allied Dunbar National Fitness Survey.* London: Sports Council & Health Education Authority.

Tolfrey, K., Jones, A. M. & Campbell, I. G. (2000) The effect of aerobic exercise training on the lipid–lipoprotein profile of children and adolescents, *Sports Medicine*, **29**, 99–112.

Tortolero, S. R., Taylor, W. C. & Murray, N. G. (2000) Physical activity, physical fitness and social, psychological and emotional health. In Armstrong, N. &

Van Mechelen, W. (eds), *Paediatric Exercise Science and Medicine*. Oxford: Oxford University Press, 273–93.

Twisk, J. W. R. (2000) Physical activity, physical fitness and cardiovascular health. In Armstrong, N. & Van Mechelen, W. (eds), *Paediatric Exercise Science and Medicine*. Oxford: Oxford University Press, 253–63.

Twisk, J. W. R., Kemper, H. C. G. & Van Mechelen, W. (2002a) The relationship between physical fitness and physical activity during adolescence and cardio-vascular disease risk factors at adult age: The Amsterdam Growth and Health Longitudinal Study, *International Journal of Sports Medicine*, **23**(supplement), S8–14.

Twisk, J. W. R., Kemper, H. C. G. & Van Mechelen, W. (2002b) Prediction of cardiovascular disease risk factors in later life by physical activity and physical fitness in youth: general comments and conclusions, *International Journal of Sports Science*, **23**(supplement), S440–50.

Welk, G. J., Corbin, C. B. & Dale, D. (2000) Measurement issues in the assessment of physical activity in children, *Research Quarterly for Exercise and Sport*, **71**(2), 59–73.

Welsman, J. & Armstrong, N. (1992) Daily physical activity and blood lactate indices of aerobic fitness, *British Journal of Sports Medicine*, **26**, 228–32.

Welsman, J. & Armstrong, N. (1996) The measurement and interpretation of aerobic fitness in children: current issues, *Journal of the Royal Society of Medicine*, **89**, 281–5.

Welsman, J. & Armstrong, N. (2000) Physical activity patterns in secondary school children, *European Physical Education Review*, **5**(2), 147–57.

Welsman, J. R., Armstrong, N., Kirby, B. J., Nevill, A. M. & Winter, E. M. (1996) Scaling peak VO_2 for differences in body size, *Medicine and Science in Sports and Exercise*, **28**, 259–65.

WHO (World Health Organization) (2000) Health and Health Behaviour Among Young People WHO Policy Series: *Health Policy for Children and Adolescents*, Issue 1, International Report. Copenhagen: WHO.

3

Monitoring Young People's Physical Fitness and Physical Activity

Lorraine Cale and Jo Harris

The measurement of both physical fitness and physical activity in young people is an important endeavour and has long been of interest to sport and exercise scientists, physical educators, and health and sports/fitness professionals. However, the problems of assessing young people's physical fitness and physical activity have been widely acknowledged (see, for example, Fox & Biddle, 1986; Armstrong, 1987; 1989; ACSM, 1988; Physical Education Association (PEA), 1988; Seefeldt & Vogel, 1989; Rowland, 1995; Cale & Harris, 1998) for physical fitness, and Melanson & Freedson, 1996; Harro & Riddoch, 2000; Kohl, Fulton & Caspersen, 2000; Rice & Howell, 2000; Welk, Corbin & Dale, 2000 for physical activity).

Monitoring techniques need to be valid, reliable and practical but, as this chapter goes on to reveal, the reliability and validity of many measures have not been established with children and adolescents. In addition, there are a number of measurement issues, some of which are generic and some of which are unique to young people, which complicate the assessment of physical fitness and physical activity. With respect to physical activity, Welk, Corbin & Dale (2000) suggest that the unique nature and characteristics of children's activity patterns (intermittent versus continuous), their less developed cognitive skills, biological differences in metabolism, and biomechanical differences in efficiency and economy can all impact upon the assessment of physical activity. The same, of course, is also true for the assessment of physical fitness.

This chapter considers the purposes and methods of monitoring physical fitness and physical activity in young people and the relative strengths and limitations of the different approaches. In particular, attention is afforded to monitoring physical activity and the practical application of physical activity assessments. This emphasis reflects the public health and exercise/physical activity promotion perspective of this book, as well as current thinking in the area which has called for a shift away from the 'product' of physical fitness and physical fitness testing, towards the 'process' of being physically active and the promotion of physical activity (Rowland, 1995; Pangrazi, 2000; Cale & Harris, 2002; Corbin, 2002). Also, many of the issues associated with physical fitness testing, including recommendations for its practical application, are addressed in detail in Chapter 9.

Monitoring physical fitness

Definition

Physical fitness has been literally and operationally defined in many ways, though typically it has been viewed as a multifactorial trait related to the capacity for movement (Pate, 1988). Caspersen, Powell & Christenson (1985) define physical fitness as a set of attributes that people have or achieve that relates to the ability to perform physical activity. In broad terms, definitions have been operationalized by identifying a list of fitness components which can be classified as health-related or performance (skill)-related (Caspersen, Powell & Christenson, 1985). The health-related components of physical fitness are related to specific 'health' or disease outcomes (Pate, 1988) and are the ones of interest here. These include cardiovascular fitness, muscular strength and endurance, flexibility and body composition (Caspersen, Powell & Christenson, 1985).

Why monitor physical fitness?

Monitoring young people's physical fitness is commonplace in school-based physical education programmes (Harris, 1995; ACSM, 2000) and is also carried out in recreational programmes, public health assessments, and in clinical settings (ACSM, 2000). Physical fitness testing in young people can serve several purposes. Within the school setting, purposes include: programme evaluation; motivation of young people; identification of children in need of improvement; identification of children with potential; screening; diagnosis of fitness needs for individual exercise prescription and improvement; the promotion of physical activity; goal setting; self-monitoring and self-testing skills; cognitive and affective learning (Whitehead, Pemberton & Corbin, 1990; Pate, 1994).

Fitness testing is also important in research. In schools, fitness data have been collected in an attempt to achieve a better understanding of fitness phenomena and their demography (Fox & Biddle, 1986). Researchers have also used fitness tests to investigate the effects of training on children's fitness. In the public health context, fitness testing has been employed in order to survey the fitness levels of young people on a large scale. National fitness surveys have been conducted in the UK, US, Canada, Australia and elsewhere to provide baseline measures from which to analyse the health-related fitness of a population. Finally, in the clinical setting, fitness testing allows for the evaluation of medical abnormalities, assessment of symptoms associated with exercise, measurement of exercise capacity, promotion of self-efficacy, and the individualization of exercise programmes (Skinner, 1993; Tomassoni, 1996; Gibbons et al., 1997).

Monitoring physical fitness in the laboratory

A brief overview of the more common laboratory-based measures of physical fitness follows. The advantages and disadvantages of these methods are summarized in Table 3.1.

Aerobic fitness

In the laboratory, the most widely used measure of cardiorespiratory fitness is maximal oxygen uptake (VO_2 max). Maximal oxygen uptake, the highest rate at which an individual can consume oxygen during exercise, limits the capacity to perform aerobic exercise and is therefore widely recognized as the best single index of aerobic fitness (Armstrong & Welsman, 1997). It is measured by collecting and analysing expired air samples during a graded, maximal exercise test, usually on a treadmill or cycle ergometer.

Table 3.1 Advantages and disadvantages of some common laboratory-based fitness tests with children

Component	Common measures	Advantages	Disadvantages
Aerobic fitness	E.g. VO_2 max	• The physiological basis for the test is well understood • Widely accepted measurement procedures exist • The test has been used as the criterion against which field measures have been validated • It has high construct validity and is highly reliable	• The test is relatively expensive and time consuming • Methods and protocols designed for adults are not always applicable to children – a special approach may be required • Achieving maximal effort can be problematic with young children
Muscular strength/endurance	*Muscular strength* Isometric dynamometer, cable tensiometer, isokinetic dynamometer, isotonic one-repetition maximum (1 R-M) tests	• Some tests (e.g. isometric strength testing via cable tensiometry or hand grip dynamometer) are relatively safe and inexpensive • Tests (e.g. isokinetic testing) can be efficient and provide specificity (e.g. isokinetic; isotonic testing) • Istonic testing provides greater joint stability and protection against injury than other testing modes	• There are generally no agreed-upon standard protocols for assessing strength in children • Some procedures (e.g. repetitive testing; 1 R-M) are not very feasible for young people

Muscular endurance
Repetitions or time to fatigue performing at a set percentage of maximum force

- Some equipment (which has been designed for adults) is costly, inappropriate and requires modification for children
- The concept and feel of tests, or the skill and experience required to perform them, is problematic for some children
- Longer habituation is recommended when employing some tests with children
- Many tests involve performing to exhaustion or some discomfort – children may not therefore be able or willing to participate

Table 3.1 (Continued)

Component	Common measures	Advantages	Disadvantages
			• The extent to which one measure of strength is an indicator of overall strength is unclear – even measures of composite strength should be viewed cautiously • The reliability of strength measures with children has not been examined extensively and few endurance tests have reliability, validity or standardization for children
Flexibility	Goniometers, the Leighton flexometer, inclinometers, tape measures	• Flexibility can be measured relatively safely, efficiently and accurately using these measures	• The cost of the equipment makes assessment prohibitive with large numbers • Flexibility is joint specific and no single test can be used to evaluate total body flexibility

| Body composition | E.g. hydrostatic weighing (or densitometry) | • Recognized as the 'gold standard' method | • Changes in chemical maturity with growth make it difficult to accurately estimate body density
• The procedure requires considerable subject co-operation (due to submersion in water)
• The technique cannot be used with very young children |

Muscular strength and muscular endurance

Though muscular strength and muscular endurance differ in concept and physiological basis, they are related and are often measured using similar or sometimes identical methods, merged into a single factor (Pate, 1991). Also, as both are specific to particular muscle groups, tests must be employed for each (Pate, 1991). Laboratory assessments of strength in children have focused predominantly on laboratory tests of isometric and isokinetic contraction strength (Armstrong & Welsman, 1997), though isotonic contraction strength testing has also been employed (Pate, 1991; Blimkie & Macauley, 2000). Blimkie & Macauley (2000) provide a detailed review and critique of the different forms of muscular strength testing with children.

In the laboratory, strength can be determined using isometric dynamometers (e.g. handgrip dynamometers) or cable tensiometers (Armstrong & Welsman, 1997), isokinetic dynamometers, or isotonic one-repetition maximum (1-RM) lift tests (i.e. the maximal resistance an individual can lift once), typically with free weights, weight-stack machines or dynamometers (Pate, 1991; Perrin, 1993). Regardless of the instrumentation, the tests involve subjects applying maximum force to an external object and strength is quantified as force applied to the isometric dynamometer, peak torque exerted against the isokinetic dynamometer, or maximum weight moved through a specified range of joint motion (Pate, 1991).

Muscular endurance can be measured using isometric, isokinetic or isotonic contractions by directing subjects to sustain an isometric contraction as long as possible at a force corresponding to a specified percentage of isometric strength, by performing isokinetic contractions at a set cadence until torque decreases to a specified percentage or maximum, or by performing the maximum number of isotonic contractions against a resistance set at a percentage of the 1-RM (Pate, 1991).

Flexibility

Just as muscular strength and endurance is specific to the muscles involved, flexibility is joint specific and no single test can be used to evaluate total body flexibility (Pate, 1991; ACSM, 2000). Laboratory tests usually quantify flexibility in terms of range of motion, expressed in degrees. Common devices for this purpose include various goniometers, electrogoniometers, the Leighton flexometer, inclinometers and tape measures (ACSM, 2000).

Body composition

Hydrostatic weighing or densitometry is the most widely used laboratory technique for assessing body composition and is recognized as the gold-standard method against which most field techniques are validated (Lohman, 1989; Boileau et al., 1986; Claessens, Beunen & Malina, 2000). The method estimates body density by measuring body weight both on land and while submerged in water, adjusted for the residual volume of air in the lungs. The derived estimate of body density is then converted to percentage body fat using a standard equation.

Monitoring physical fitness in the field

Physical fitness testing in the field typically involves the administration of a battery of simple tests to evaluate different components of fitness (ACSM, 2000). A number of such tests are commonly employed with young people and a summary of the most popular is provided here and in Table 3.2. In addition, a specific and general critique of the tests and test batteries is presented.

Aerobic fitness/capacity

Distance runs have been the most commonly used field measures with children (Pate, 1991). The mile run/walk in which children complete the distance as quickly as possible has been included in several fitness test batteries (e.g. AAHPERD, FITNESSGRAM). Other variations include the 1.5-mile run, or the 9- or 12-minute run for distance. Several factors, however, affect children's performance of the distance run, including their economy of gait, experience, motor efficiency, environmental conditions and motivation (Safrit, 1990), and the relevance and appropriateness of the mile run test for children has been questioned (Hopple & Graham, 1995). Also, the reliability of various distance run tests has been reported to be high, but not uniformly so, and the need for additional investigations of the reliability and validity of the tests has been identified (Safrit, 1990).

More recently the Multistage Fitness Test has assumed popularity (Brewer, Ramsbottom & Williams, 1988; 2001). The test, also referred to as the 'bleep' test, is a progressive shuttle-run test for the prediction of maximum oxygen uptake (Eve & Williams, 2000). Promoters claim that the Multistage Fitness Test provides a relatively straightforward

Table 3.2 A summary of some of the more common field tests of physical fitness for children

Component	Measurement procedures
Aerobic fitness/capacity	Distance/timed walks/runs (1, 1.5 mile; 9-, 12-minute) Step tests Multistage Fitness Test
Muscular strength/endurance	Sit ups/curl ups Progressive abdominal sit-up (curl) test Pull-ups Modified pull-ups Push-ups
Flexibility	Sit and reach Shoulder stretch Arm lift
Body composition	Body mass index (BMI) Skinfold thicknesses Girth measures
Agility*	Shuttle run Dodging runs
Anaerobic power*	Standing broad jump Vertical jump Sprints

* Anaerobic power and agility are not health-related components of fitness but are still commonly employed in field test batteries.

means of monitoring aerobic fitness with young people in a practical way, without the need or use of sophisticated scientific equipment and measuring devices (Eve & Williams, 2000). However, written pre-test precautions provided with the test indicate the need for maximal effort if the result is to be valid (Eve & Williams, 2000). In this and other respects, the appropriateness of the test for use with young people has been questioned (Cale & Harris, 2002). The test was developed for use with elite, adult populations and is often applied to young people with little consideration of the differences between children's and adults' responses to exercise. Indeed, risks associated with using the Multi-stage Fitness Test with young people have been identified recently and safety advice has been given on how to reduce such risks (Eve & Williams, 2000).

Muscular strength and muscular endurance

Field tests of muscular fitness traditionally involve resisting or moving part or all of the body mass (Armstrong & Welsman, 1997). The abdominal region and upper arm girdle musculatures have received greatest attention in testing, and common exercises include sit-ups or curl-ups, pull-ups and flexed arm-hangs (Pate & Shephard, 1989; Pate, 1991). The tests usually involve performing as many repetitions of the exercise as possible in a specified time or before reaching exhaustion. More recently however, a 'progressive abdominal sit-up test' which involves performing the curl-up in time to a controlled and timed 'bleep' until the subject can no longer continue has been developed (Brewer & Davis, 2000). For most youngsters (i.e. those who can perform more than one repetition), the tests rely predominantly on muscular endurance rather than strength, and are therefore usually described as measures of muscular strength/endurance (Pate, 1991).

In the sit-up test for the abdominals, a variety of leg muscles and the hip flexors contribute to the movement, the involvement of the latter of which can have a negative impact on the lower back (Safrit, 1990). The curl-up, involving a smaller range of movement, was therefore proposed as an alternative for maximal involvement of the abdominals. Both tests, however, have face validity in that the abdominals are used during the tests (Pate, 1991) and both are considered to be moderately reliable (Safrit, 1990).

Performance on the pull-up test is confounded by body weight and many youngsters are unable to perform one repetition (Ross & Gilbert, 1985; Pate et al., 1987). Not surprisingly, very good reliability has been reported for the test but its validity is open to question (Safrit, 1990). In response, modified versions of the test have been developed (Pate et al., 1987) which have shown good reliability and have discriminated well among subjects (Safrit, 1990).

Flexibility

Because poor flexibility in the lower back and hamstring region is considered a cause of lower-back pain, common field tests involve assessing the range of motion at the hip joint (Pate, 1991). By far the most common test is the sit and reach. Others include the shoulder stretch (Cooper Institute for Aerobics Research, 1999) or the arm lift (Corbin & Lindsey, 2002). Most tests, however, only measure part of the range of motion (Docherty, 1996). Also, whilst the sit and reach is considered a reliable test, fewer validation studies have been carried out (Pate, 1991) and validity and reliability data for other tests are lacking.

Body composition

In the field, body composition is typically estimated using anthropometry (Pate, 1991). Stature-mass indices such as the body mass index (BMI) have been widely employed (Kemper, 1985), though the use of skinfold thicknesses is the most common technique and provides a useful indicator of young people's subcutaneous fatness (Armstrong & Welsman, 1997; Claessens, Beunen & Malina, 2000). Skinfolds are usually taken from a few selected sites of the body (commonly the triceps, biceps, subscapular, suprailiac, front thigh and medial calf in young people). The sum of the skinfolds can be used as an indication of total body fat or can be entered into a regression equation to predict either body density and/or percentage body fat (Claessens, Beunen & Malina, 2000). Skinfolds are relatively easy and inexpensive to obtain and provide a relatively simple and non-invasive method of estimating general fatness (Claessens, Beunen & Malina, 2000). The method has also been found to correlate well with other measures (e.g. hydrostatic weight) (Lohman, 1989).

The technique does have limitations however. The relationship between skinfolds and body fatness, as estimated from body density, varies with maturity status which precludes the accurate prediction of young people's total body fatness from skinfold measures (Lohman, Boileau & Slaughter, 1984). Prediction equations which account for age, gender and maturational stage have been developed (Slaughter et al., 1988) and received support (Janz et al., 1993; Lohman, 1992), though further research is required to explore their validity (Armstrong & Welsman, 1997). Finally, consideration must also be given to the large inter-observer variability typically associated with skinfold measurements (Armstrong & Welsman, 1997).

Physical fitness test batteries

Some schools, communities and surveys develop their own tests, test batteries and standards of performance to assess physical fitness

(Ross, 1989). However, a number of formal fitness test batteries have been developed over the years. The first battery to be widely used was the American Alliance for Health, Physical Education, and Recreation Youth Fitness Test (AAHPER, 1976) (Fox & Biddle, 1986; Pate, 1994) which was developed in the United States. However, despite several revisions, the test was labelled throughout as a test of motor fitness, and subsequently faced criticism and lost popularity (Pate, 1994). Thus, by the late 1980s other fitness testing programmes were developed in the United States which more closely reflected the contemporary thinking concerning approaches to fitness measurement in young people (Pate, 1994). Examples include AAHPERD's Physical Best (which replaced the Youth Fitness Test and is now a comprehensive fitness education programme), the Chrylser/AAU Test, FITNESSGRAM, the National Children and Youth Fitness Study, the Presidential Physical Fitness Award and the YMCA Youth Fitness Test. In addition, test batteries have also been developed in Canada, Australia, Europe and elsewhere (Fox & Biddle, 1986).

Not surprisingly, the major batteries have a number of similarities and are more alike than they are different (Safrit, 1990; Pate, 1994). They all emphasize and measure common components of health-related fitness and many contain the same or similar tests (Safrit, 1990). More recently, the fourth revision of FITNESSGRAM (Cooper Institute for Aerobics Research, 1999), has perhaps become the most established and well-known battery. FITNESSGRAM is a comprehensive health-related fitness and activity assessment and computerized reporting system (Cooper Institute for Aerobics Research, 1999). Its goals are to promote enjoyable regular physical activity and to provide comprehensive physical fitness and activity assessments and reporting programmes for children and youth. The programme is designed to evaluate and educate young people about their physical fitness and includes various components of fitness, with several test options provided for most areas and one recommended test item. These include measures and tests of aerobic fitness (e.g. the PACER (a progressive endurance run); one mile run), body composition (skinfold measurements; body mass index), muscular strength, endurance and flexibility (e.g. curl-up; push-up; pull-up) and flexibility (e.g. sit and reach; shoulder stretch).

FITNESSGRAM uses criterion-referenced standards to evaluate performance, which is classified in two general categories, 'Needs improvement' and 'Healthy Fitness Zone'. The report generates personalized output and recommendations based on the results. Additional features include a physical activity assessment and a recognition programme 'You Stay Active'.

General critique of fitness tests and fitness test batteries

As can be seen from the overview of the individual test items, each has merits as well as limitations. In addition, there are advantages and disadvantages which are common to a number of the tests and to fitness test batteries in general. As mentioned previously, fitness tests can potentially serve several useful purposes. Field tests are also generally easy to administer, time-efficient, relatively safe and involve minimal equipment and low cost. According to Safrit (1990), advances in the development and use of physical fitness tests for children have been impressive. Considerable thought has been given to the scientific evidence supporting a test, and the emphasis is now clearly on the evaluation of health-related fitness components (Pate, 1994). Also the emphasis has shifted in recent years from testing in isolation, to an educational programme with testing as an integral part. Physical fitness programmes are now packaged attractively and include test manuals, curricular guidelines and instructional materials to assist the user/teacher (Safrit, 1990; Pate, 1994). Some also have computerized feedback systems.

Standards of performance are identified by the fitness test programmes and often linked to award or recognition systems (Safrit, 1990). Several of the major test batteries have also developed criterion-referenced standards for interpreting results (Cureton & Warren, 1990). These are absolute standards that specify the minimum levels of fitness thought to be required for health and to perform daily tasks. Despite their limitations (described below), criterion-referenced standards are attractive from a theoretical standpoint in that they communicate to young people that there is a level of fitness (below that needed to be a successful athlete) that is satisfactory for health maintenance (Pate, 1994) and they categorize individuals into groups that either meet or exceed the minimum standards and those that do not (Cureton, 1994). As such, they are favoured over the use of normative standards, which involve the comparison of a child's score with that of a reference group.

Advances in the development and use of fitness tests for children have undoubtedly been made in recent years, yet a number of issues and concerns remain. The discussion here, however, concerns itself only with those issues that are directly related to the measurement of physical fitness and the measures themselves. (See Chapter 9 for a general discussion of fitness testing in young people, including issues relating to the promotion of physical activity.)

As is evident from the previous section, the appropriateness, validity and reliability of some fitness tests (including laboratory- and field-based) for use with children is questionable (Safrit, 1990; Safrit & Looney, 1992; Rowland, 1995; Rice & Howell, 2000). It is generally accepted that field tests provide only a crude measure of an individual's physical fitness. As highlighted earlier, the appropriateness of some tests for children (e.g. the Multistage Fitness Test) is doubtful in that they have been developed for use with elite, adult populations; a child's metabolic, cardiopulmonary, thermoregulatory and perceptual responses to exercise are different from those of adults and a special approach may therefore be required in administering tests to children (Bar-Or, 1993).

Problems with the validity and reliability of some commonly used fitness tests with children and the need for additional evidence of the reliability and validity of tests and test batteries have been identified (Safrit, 1990). Safrit (1990) notes how the reliability of individual tests has usually been assumed to be high because the subject is expected to put maximum effort into the test, but in reality maximum effort is not always exerted. Furthermore, the reliability of a total test battery has seldom been examined (Safrit, 1990). On the issue of validity, some tests (e.g. pull-ups, sit and reach) present more of a concern than others. Furthermore, the validity of tests cannot automatically be generalized across age groups (Safrit, 1990). The PEA (1988) claim that several of the more popular field tests are not even based on sound physiological foundations and that many of the data generated by fitness tests are therefore problematic and not capable of rigorous interpretation.

The problems of validity and reliability are perhaps better understood when one considers the many factors that influence performance on fitness tests (both laboratory- and field-based). Fitness test scores are a result in all cases of the weighted contribution of a number of factors which are probably somewhat related (Fox & Biddle, 1986). Factors such as the environment/test conditions (e.g. temperature, humidity, wind speed/direction), lifestyle (exercise/nutrition), test protocol/procedures, motivation, intellectual and mechanical skill at taking the test, heredity or genetic potential, and maturation all affect fitness performance and will be reflected in fitness test scores (Fox & Biddle, 1986; Docherty & Bell, 1990; Pangrazi, 2000). The relative contribution of these factors varies from test to test, and between testing sessions (Fox & Biddle, 1986), though heredity or genetic potential and maturation are considered to most strongly influence test results (Pangrazi & Corbin, 1990; Bouchard et al., 1992). Within a given age group of early adolescents, there will be large variation in maturation level and associated variations in size will influence performance. During this time, young people may experience an increase or decrease in their ability to perform certain test items, independent of their fitness. In general, more mature youngsters usually perform better on tests than the less mature. However, early-maturing girls may be disadvantaged in some tests (e.g. in tests of aerobic capacity such as the distance run or tests in which the body must be lifted or moved, such as pull-ups) because of the increase in body fat and other physical changes which accompany puberty (Fox & Biddle, 1986; Docherty & Bell, 1990). Armstrong (1995) and Armstrong & Biddle (1992) recognize the importance of both maturation and motivation to test scores and claim that fitness tests simply determine the obvious, at best only distinguishing the mature and/or motivated from the immature and/or unmotivated.

Concerning heredity or genetic potential, health-related fitness tests have a clear genetic component, and some young people will be advantaged on tests because of the physical characteristics they inherit (Fox & Biddle, 1986; Bouchard, 1993). The anatomical and physiological features which seem to stand out in importance include size and morphology of the heart and circulatory system, muscle fibre typing, sensitivity to training or 'trainability', and somatotype and body size (Fox & Biddle, 1986).

The practice of applying norm and/or criterion-referenced standards in fitness testing also has limitations. For example, norm tables do not indicate desired levels of physical fitness or provide any diagnostic feedback, and they imply that 'more is better' (Cureton, 1994). Armstrong & Welsman (1997) also report how the use of norm tables promotes ego-orientation and confounds the issue of relative fitness because tables constructed on the basis of chronological age cannot be used to classify legitimately young people at different levels of maturity. With criterion-referenced standards, it could be argued that, because they represent desired minimum levels of fitness, they do not provide an incentive to young people to achieve higher fitness levels (Cureton, 1994). There is also no evidence on the validity of criterion-referenced standards with young people, and it is not always clear how standards have been determined (Docherty & Bell, 1990; Safrit, 1990) and the extent to which they have been established arbitrarily (Cureton, 1994). It is also of concern that standards developed for the same test items on different youth fitness tests often differ quite considerably (e.g. by as much as three minutes on some tests) (Safrit, 1990; Cureton, 1994). Furthermore, the use of arbitrary criterion-referenced standards could lead to misclassifications of fitness level, which could have negative consequences for the individual concerned. Indeed, following a review of the validity and reliability of fitness tests for children, Safrit (1990) suggested that additional evidence of the validity and reliability of test batteries, including test items, criterion-referenced standards and national norms was required.

In summary, there are clearly a number of issues and limitations concerning the measurement of physical fitness in young people and, in the words of Safrit (1990, p. 25), it would seem that 'much still needs to be done' to improve the validity, reliability, practicality and thereby utility of fitness testing in young people. In light of this, the issue of the practical application of monitoring physical fitness is now raised (see discussion point below) and pursued further in Chapter 9.

Discussion point

- How might the following groups employ physical fitness tests with young people and use the fitness test data?

  - researchers
  - physical education teachers
  - health practitioners
  - sports coaches
  - exercise instructors

- What considerations would each group need to take into account in choosing which measures of physical fitness to employ?
- In your view, what represents good fitness testing practice with young people?
- What additional considerations should be taken into account when monitoring physical fitness in young people?

Monitoring physical activity

Definition

Physical activity is a complex behaviour that incorporates all the activities of daily living (Cooper, 2003). Conventionally, it is defined as any bodily movement produced by skeletal muscles that results in energy expenditure (Caspersen, Powell & Christenson, 1985). It has dimensions of volume (how much), duration (how long), frequency (how often), intensity (how hard) and mode (what type). In addition, the many diverse areas of everyday physical activity – exercise, sport, recreation, occupational activity, non-occupational activity – need to be accounted for when considering activity (Cooper, 2003).

Why monitor physical activity?

The measurement of physical activity in young people has become an important field of interest for a number of reasons. For the purposes of research, the accurate assessment of physical activity in young people is necessary for determining current levels of physical activity, monitoring compliance with physical activity guidelines, determining the effectiveness of intervention programmes designed to improve physical activity, and understanding the dose–response relationship between physical activity and health (Sirard & Pate, 2001). From an educational and exercise/ physical activity promotion perspective, and perhaps with the exception of understanding the dose–response relationship, these purposes are also relevant. In addition, and with reference specifically to PE, Cale (1998) and Welk & Wood (2000) suggest a variety of uses for activity monitoring which are outlined at the end of this chapter.

Methods of monitoring physical activity

More than thirty different methods of assessing physical activity have been identified (Melanson & Freedson, 1996; Armstrong & Welsman, 1997). Within reviews, the various methods tend to be classified into different measurement categories. For example, Sirard & Pate (2001) identify three types of measures of physical activity in children and adolescents, primary (e.g. observation, doubly-labelled water and indirect calorimetry); secondary (e.g. heart rate monitors, pedometers and accelerometers); and subjective (e.g. self-report), and Kohl, Fulton & Caspersen (2000) identify six categories of techniques (self-report, electronic or mechanical monitoring, observation, indirect calorimetry, doubly-labelled water, and direct calorimetry). Armstrong & Welsman (1997) group the techniques into the four categories that are outlined below.

Self- and/or proxy report

Self-report is probably the most commonly used measure of young people's physical activity (Sallis, 1991). The types of self-report measure employed with young people include self-report questionnaires, interviewer-administered questionnaires, diaries and proxy reports (in which parents or teachers report the child's activity using any of the other formats) (Sallis, 1991; Sirard & Pate, 2001). Measures vary in the specificity with which mode, duration, intensity and frequency of physical activity are assessed, in the period of time covered by the report, and in whether the data are reported as ratings, activity scores, times, calories expended, or other summary scores (Sallis, 1991). In recent years a variety of self-report measures have been developed for use with children (see Welk & Wood, 2000), two of which are presented in the following section.

Self-report instruments provide a convenient way to assess activity patterns in large populations (Welk, Corbin & Dale, 2000). They are convenient/quick to administer, involve low investigator and respondent burden, and are cost-effective, unobtrusive and non-reactive when compared to other measures (Baranowski, 1988; Sallis, 1991; Armstrong & Welsman, 1997; Welk & Wood, 2000; Sirard & Pate, 2001). Self-reports are also versatile and may cover details of activity for the previous days, weeks, months or even years, and can be used to measure a variety of physical activity variables from one source (Cale, 1994). In addition, the recent development and use of computerized questionnaires (e.g. the Computer Delivered Physical Activity Questionnaire (CDPAQ) (Ridley, Dollman & Olds, 2001) and ACTIVITYGRAM (Cooper Institute for Aerobics Research, 1999) offer promise to assist with recall and coding of activity (Welk, Corbin & Dale, 2000) and have enormous time-saving potential (Ridley, Dollman & Olds, 2001).

However, concern has been expressed over the accuracy of self-report data obtained from children (Welk, Corbin & Dale, 2000). Reviews of validity and reliability studies of measurement techniques conducted with children have concluded that self-report methods are reasonably reliable but have lower validity (Harro & Riddoch, 2000; Kohl, Fulton & Caspersen, 2000). Self-reports are subjective measures because they rely on responses from the child (Sirard & Pate, 2001) and actual behaviour is not directly assessed via this method (Armstrong & Welsman, 1997). As a consequence, issues of recall errors, interpretation, deliberate mis-representations, social desirability and other biases are important (Sirard & Pate, 2001). In particular, children's lower cognitive ability compared with adults reduces their ability to accurately recall frequency, intensity and especially duration of activities, as many youngsters do not wear watches, or may be less time-conscious or ill-equipped to tell or estimate time (Baranowski et al., 1984; Baranowski, 1988; Sallis, 1991). Also, the sporadic nature and intensity of their activity makes it difficult to recall, quantify and categorize (Harro & Riddoch, 2000; Sirard & Pate, 2001). It has also been suggested that questionnaires are likely to be inappropriate for activity which is unstructured (i.e. play time), which is a frequent source of activity for young people (Kohl, Fulton & Caspersen, 2000).

The extent to which self-report measures are affected by such problems varies and depends on the type of measure and on the age and development level of the children to which the measure is applied. Self-report measures are not considered useful with children under 10–12 years of age (Sallis, 1991; Pate, 1993; Harro & Riddoch, 2000; Kohl, Fulton & Caspersen, 2000). However, by the time young people reach high school they are reported to become cognitively and behaviourally more similar to adults (Welk, Corbin & Dale, 2000). The consensus from several reviews is that previous-day recall instruments offer the most promise with children (Welk, Corbin & Dale, 2000). Self-administered questionnaires are considered to be less accurate than interviewer-administered questionnaires, and diaries are considered to be superior to retrospective questionnaires (Armstrong & Welsman, 1997). However, memory recall can be enhanced through memory cues (Baranowski, 1988), for example structuring questionnaires to provide time-related cues (e.g. before school, during school, after school), separating weekday and weekend activity, or providing checklists of common activities.

Physiological analyses

Indirect calorimetry

Indirect calorimetry and doubly-labelled water (described below) are recognized to be the respective gold standard assessments for studies on physical activity (Welk, Corbin & Dale, 2000; Sirard & Pate, 2001). Indirect calorimetry measures energy expenditure from oxygen consumption and carbon dioxide production to provide accurate minute-by-minute measurements. However, because the measure involves analysing expired air, it requires cumbersome equipment and subjects to wear a facemask or a mouthpiece and noseclip (Armstrong & Welsman, 1997; Sirard & Pate, 2001), which interferes with normal daily activities (Cooper, 2003). The technique is therefore considered unsuitable for assessing young people's physical activity (Armstrong & Welsman, 1997; Sirard & Pate, 2001).

Doubly-labelled water technique

This technique uses the stable (non-radioactive) isotopes deuterium ($^2H_2$) and ^{18}O and is considered to be the most accurate method for measuring total energy expenditure in free-living individuals (Cooper, 2003). Cooper (2003) provides a useful summary of the technique but, briefly, an oral dose of water enriched with deuterium and ^{18}O is given and sequential urine samples are taken over a period of days to monitor the disappearance of the isotopes from the body. The rate of isotope disappearance depends upon the individual's level of physical activity.

Doubly-labelled water is advantageous in that it can be used easily in free living and does not interfere with normal activity patterns, activity can be measured over one to two weeks without constant supervision, and it has low reactivity (Kohl, Fulton & Caspersen, 2000; Welk, Corbin & Dale, 2000; Sirard & Pate, 2001). Furthermore, the accuracy, subject simplicity and non-invasive nature of the method make it an ideal and promising field technique in children (Schoeller, 1983; Saris, 1985). There are, however, limitations with doubly-labelled water. The isotopes are difficult to obtain, hence expensive, the collection of multiple urine samples and laboratory visits is burdensome, and the analysis of samples is a complex and expensive task. The method is not therefore suitable for large studies (Kohl, Fulton & Caspersen, 2000; Sirard & Pate, 2001). Also, the data provide only a measure of total energy expenditure over the study period; types and activity patterns are not investigated (Armstrong & Van Mechelen, 1998; Kohl, Fulton & Caspersen, 2000; Sirard & Pate, 2001).

Heart rate monitoring

In comparison with other physiological measures, heart rate monitoring is considered the most suitable single method for use in large-scale physical activity studies with children (Saris, 1985; Emons et al., 1992; Livingstone et al., 1992). Given the strong association between heart rate and energy expenditure during exercise, it has frequently been used to estimate daily activity in children as a sole criterion, and to validate other methods (Eston, Rowlands & Ingledew, 1998). A number of self-contained, computerized telemetry systems have been developed which typically consist of a lightweight transmitter, fixed to the chest with electrodes, and a receiver/microcomputer which is worn as a wristwatch (Armstrong & Welsman, 1997).

Heart rate monitoring has a number of advantages. Monitors are small, relatively cheap and robust, and are designed to function under many conditions, including during water-based activities (Cooper, 2003). The latest systems can record information for periods of between 22 and

260 hours. Furthermore, the method is easy to use, unobtrusive, socially acceptable, permits freedom of movement and, because monitors are not immediately noticeable, they should not unduly influence children's normal activity patterns (Armstrong & Welsman, 1997). Heart rate monitoring is also generally accepted as a reliable and valid physiological quantification of activity (Armstrong, 1998) and instruments have been found to be reliable and valid with young people (Treiber et al., 1989; Durant et al., 1993).

Heart rate, however, does not measure activity directly, but the individual's physiological response to activity (Cooper, 2003). Yet many factors besides physical activity can influence heart rate, with differential effects on oxygen requirement (Rowlands, Eston & Ingledew, 1997; Harro & Riddoch, 2000). For example, the metabolism of the individual, emotional stress, anxiety, fatigue, state of hydration, food intake, ambient temperature and humidity, body position, posture, active muscle group, type of muscle contraction, type of exercise, and training status or fitness level (Melanson & Freedson, 1996; Rowlands, Eston & Ingledew, 1997; Armstrong & Van Mechelen, 1998; Eston, Rowlands & Ingledew, 1998; Harro & Riddoch, 2000; Welk, Corbin & Dale, 2000). These are all potential sources of error which make the interpretation of heart rate data complex. Eston, Rowlands & Ingledew (1998) also suggest that the relative delay in heart rate response to changes in movement may mask information, and equally the heart rate possibly remaining elevated after VO_2 has returned to normal may result in an overestimation of energy expenditure. Other issues include problems with interference and lost data from signal interruptions (Harro & Riddoch, 2000; Welk, Corbin & Dale, 2000), and discomfort from wearing the transmitter, which can reduce participant compliance (Welk, Corbin & Dale, 2000).

Finally, there is no consensus on the most appropriate method for summarizing heart rate data (Harro & Riddoch, 2000). A number of investigators have reported the total or percentage time the heart rate is above a certain criterion (e.g. time spent in moderate to vigorous physical activity), or noted the number and length of sustained periods above threshold levels (Armstrong & Van Mechelen, 1998). Others have predicted young people's energy expenditure from the heart rate data (Verschuur & Kemper, 1985; Saris, 1986; Riddoch et al., 1991) though this methodology is problematic and should be interpreted cautiously (Armstrong & Van Mechelen, 1998).

Motion-sensor monitoring

Movement counters

The simplest form of motion sensor is the pedometer (often called step counter), which provides an objective indicator of step counts, a marker of total volume or duration of physical activity (Welk, Corbin & Dale, 2000). The pedometer can also provide an estimate of the distance walked by incorporating a measure of stride length, and some can provide a crude estimate of energy expenditure if body weight is incorporated (Cooper, 2003). It is generally worn on the hip/waist and relies on vertical movements of the body to trigger a switch (mechanical or electrical) each time a step is taken.

The main advantages of pedometers are that they are small, inexpensive, unobtrusive, non-reactive, objective and reusable (Sirard & Pate, 2001; Cooper, 2003). As a result, they appear to be well-suited to measuring physical activity in children (Rowlands, Eston & Ingledew, 1997; Cooper, 2003). Pedometers, though, are limited in the nature of the activity information they provide. For example, they do not provide any temporal information about activity patterns (Cooper, 2003) and they do not measure intensity of activity (Rowlands, Eston & Ingledew, 1997). Furthermore, pedometers are not very sensitive to physical activity that does not involve locomotion or impact (e.g. skateboarding), or that involves the upper body (e.g. throwing/catching), and they do not account for increases in energy expenditure due to carrying objects or walking/running uphill (Rowlands, Eston & Ingledew, 1997; Cooper, 2003). In the past, pedometers have been considered inaccurate and unreliable (Rowlands, Eston & Ingledew, 1997) though recent advances in technology have led to increased reliability and validity (Bassett, Ainsworth & Leggett, 1996; Bassett et al., 2000).

Accelerometers

Accelerometers are more sophisticated electronic devices that measure accelerations produced by body movement. They are also usually worn on the hip but use piezo-electric transducers and microprocessors to convert body accelerations to a quantifiable digital signal referred to as counts (Sirard & Pate, 2001). A number of accelerometers are available that range in complexity and cost (e.g. the Caltrac, a single (vertical) plane accelerometer, and the Tritrac, a three-dimensional device). The review of reliability and validity studies by Kohl, Fulton & Caspersen

(2000) suggests moderate to high reliability of such monitoring methods but low to moderate validity.

Accelerometers provide an objective, non-reactive, relatively unobtrusive, and reusable tool for assessing physical activity (Sirard & Pate, 2001). They measure quantity and intensity of movement, and the more sophisticated devices such as the Tritrac have a time-sampling mechanism that allows a chronological measure of frequency, intensity and duration of movement. They can also store data over many days (Rowlands, Eston & Ingledew, 1997). Limitations of accelerometers are their inability to assess upper-body activities (Welk, Corbin & Dale, 2000) and their limited ability to assess cycling and locomotion on a gradient (Sirard & Pate, 2001). Also, as a single-plane accelerometer, the Caltrac is limited in its ability to detect the wide variety of movements engaged in by young people (Sirard & Pate, 2001) and the sporadic nature of their activity patterns may not be adequately represented (Sallis et al., 1990). It is also unable to detect daily or hourly patterns of activity (Freedson, 1991; Rowlands, Eston & Ingledew, 1997; Sirard & Pate, 2001). The Tritrac overcomes some of these limitations. Finally, although both devices can be programmed to provide an estimate of energy expenditure, the methodology makes a number of unsubstantiated assumptions and may provide inaccurate estimates (Armstrong & Van Mechelen, 1998; Sirard & Pate, 2001). It is therefore advisable to use activity counts as the criterion measure (Freedson, 1991; Pate, 1993).

Observation

Observation involves witnessing physical activity behaviour while recording it on a coding form or through a handheld computer device (Pate, 1993), and converting the data into some type of summary score (Kohl, Fulton & Caspersen, 2000). Observation techniques are considered well-suited to children and to provide one of the best criterion measures to validate other assessment tools (Welk, Corbin & Dale, 2000). Physical activity is assessed directly through observation, and technological advances permitting complex observational codes to be entered, stored and analysed by portable computers make this method appealing (McKenzie, 1991). Various instruments for the systematic observation of young people's physical activity have been developed for use in school/PE (e.g. the Children's Physical Activity Form (CPAF)) (O'Hara et al., 1989), as well as in general settings (e.g. the Children's Activity Rating Scale (CARS) (Puhl et al., 1990)) and are reviewed elsewhere (McKenzie, 1991; Sirard & Pate, 2001).

Measures can yield accurate and detailed data on different dimensions of activity (Harro & Riddoch, 2000). In addition, they allow brief periods and sudden changes in activity to be captured, which is crucial to the study of children (Sirard & Pate, 2001). Furthermore, young people's activity levels can be observed reliably and observers can quickly be trained to record accurate information (Armstrong & Welsman, 1997).

McKenzie (1991), however, identifies a number of disadvantages with observation. For example, events studied must be observable and codable and are therefore limited to events seen or heard, and observers need to be present during the observation, thereby limiting the situations where data can be collected. Other drawbacks are the relatively high experimenter burden with conducting observations and the potential reactivity of the subjects (Sirard & Pate, 2001). Considerable time and energy is required to develop the observational system, prepare coding conventions, and train observers. Furthermore, the total observation time required to attain acceptable day-to-day stability is not clear for most instruments (Sirard & Pate, 2001). The above factors make observation labour-intensive, time-consuming and therefore costly in comparison to other methods (McKenzie, 1991; Armstrong & Welsman, 1997).

The practical application of monitoring physical activity

Evidently, then, there are a number of different measures to choose from when monitoring young people's physical activity. The ideal method, however, remains elusive (Sirard & Pate, 2001) as each has strengths and weaknesses (Kohl, Fulton & Caspersen, 2000). According to Welk, Corbin & Dale (2000), the inherent limitations of each method, along with the nature of children's movement patterns and the various types of activities engaged in, limit the ultimate accuracy of all measurements. In selecting and employing any measure, though, the advantages and disadvantages must be considered as well as the purpose of the assessment and the age of the participants, which will vary both between and within different contexts. Here a distinction is made between the assessment of physical activity for the purposes of research versus that for educational outcomes and/or exercise/physical activity promotion.

Research

In the research setting, selection of an instrument depends on the specific research question being addressed, as well as the relative importance of accuracy and practicality (Baranowski & Simons-Morton, 1988). Relatively weak measures are probably sufficient to demonstrate general health benefits of physical activity, but more sophisticated techniques are needed to answer more complex research questions and would be of use in aetiological studies, in tracking trends in physical activity, in making objective comparisons between populations, and in monitoring the effect of interventions (Wareham & Rennie, 1998).

Selecting a measure involves an accuracy–practicality trade-off, which presents a more challenging predicament with children than it does with adults (Welk, Corbin & Dale, 2000). With young people, an instrument must be sensitive enough to record sporadic and intermittent activity (Welk, Corbin & Dale, 2000).

Based on a review of the available literature, Saris (1985) summarized the most suitable methods of measuring physical activity in children depending on the number of subjects. For numbers of more than a hundred, he advocated the use of questionnaire or movement counter, for between 20 and 100, he recommended heart rate monitoring or movement counters, and for fewer than 20, doubly-labelled water, heart rate monitoring, indirect calorimetry or observation. More recently, Harro & Riddoch (2000) have provided a summary of how various assessment methods compare in children taking into account factors including validity, cost, objectivity, ease of administration, ease of completion, dimensions of activity assessed, reactivity, feasibility for large-scale studies, and suitability for younger and older children. They conclude that heart rate monitoring and motion sensors display an optimum balance of all features.

Finally, given that there seems to be no single 'best' method for monitoring physical activity and all have deficiencies and are not measuring identical properties or components, a number of researchers have recommended using a combination of, or multiple, methods (Saris, 1985; 1986; Armstrong & Welsman, 1997; Kohl, Fulton & Caspersen, 2000; Welk, Corbin & Dale, 2000). Welk, Corbin & Dale, (2000) suggest that employing multiple measures may help better to characterize young people's activity levels, provide a more complete description of their activity, and permit a triangulation of outcomes. Armstrong & Welsman (1997) and Armstrong & Van Mechelen (1998) identify the following combination of methods to evaluate young people's activity: (1) observation to note frequency, duration and type of activity, (2) heart rate monitoring to note patterns of relative physiological load (intensity) on the cardio-pulmonary system, and (3) doubly-labelled water to note total energy expenditure.

Education and exercise/physical activity promotion

To date, the importance and use of monitoring young people's physical activity in practical settings, and how educationalists, and health and other professionals might approach this has been given relatively little attention. Rice & Howell (2000) have considered the implications of the measurement of physical activity and physical fitness for health care practitioners, and others (Harris & Elbourn, 1994; Cale, 1998; Welk & Wood, 2000) have considered physical activity monitoring in the educational context. Welk & Wood (2000) note how, if the promotion of physical activity is an appropriate behavioural target for PE, then at least some emphasis should be placed on assessing physical activity in the curriculum.

Cale (1998) identified a number of reasons why teachers should monitor young people's activity. Firstly, the promotion of physical activity in young people should involve establishing how active they are and whether they are meeting current physical activity guidelines for young people (see Chapter 5). This entails monitoring activity levels. Secondly, monitoring physical activity relates to the National Curriculum for Physical Education (NCPE) requirements. Harris (2000) presents an interpretation of the health and fitness requirements of the NCPE expressed in the form of learning outcomes for each Key Stage (see Chapter 7). Clearly, to establish whether young people have achieved some of these (e.g. at Key Stage 3, pupils should 'participate in activity of at least moderate intensity…preferably for one hour every day' (p. 38)) requires informed assessments of their activity behaviour. Finally, calls have been made for the profession to focus more on physical activity behaviour as a desirable outcome of physical activity promotion and health-related PE programmes than on fitness (Harris & Cale, 1997; Pangrazi, 2000; Cale & Harris, 2002; Corbin, 2002) (see Chapter 9).

When choosing a measure of physical activity for use within an educational or exercise/physical activity promotion context, the extremes of accuracy often sought by researchers are not usually required. For example, factors such as cost, ease of use, and educational value should probably be weighed more heavily (Welk & Wood, 2000). Such constraints may influence the accuracy of the data collected but they need not necessarily detract from the value of the assessment. Welk & Wood (2000) suggest that, rather than worrying about the precision of the evaluation, it is more important to ensure that young people learn something from the process. Indeed, Cale (1998) and Welk & Wood (2000) have identified those measures that are deemed feasible for use with young people in schools and present ideas as to how these might be incorporated within PE. Their ideas, which are considered equally applicable to health and other practitioners, are summarized below.

Observation

Valuable information can be gathered from observation without having to employ sophisticated techniques. Simple observation sheets could be prepared on which all details of activity could be recorded. Children could be asked to observe and record the physical activity behaviour of a peer during a school day or week, which would involve tracking the individual's movements during lessons, break-times, lunchtimes and after school.

Heart rate monitoring

Heart rate monitors have frequently been used in the PE curriculum to help young people learn about the cardiovascular system and target heart ranges (Welk & Wood, 2000). Cost is likely to prohibit the purchase of multiple heart rate monitors, and therefore collecting data on large numbers, but one or two monitors could be used effectively within PE (Cale, 1998). Selected individuals could monitor their heart rate during lessons, a school day, or over a more extended period of time (e.g. a school week; a unit of work) and the data shared and discussed.

Motion sensors

As with heart rate monitors, cost is likely to be an issue with many motion sensors. Pedometers, however, are now reasonably affordable and could be used with young people in much the same way as heart rate monitors (Cale, 1998).

Self-report

Self-report instruments probably offer the greatest potential for use in the curriculum (Welk & Wood, 2000) and are likely to be the most practical and useful method of monitoring activity in the field. An existing questionnaire could be adopted to meet particular needs (Welk & Wood, 2000) or an alternative questionnaire could be developed, perhaps using existing forms as a guide. Two example questionnaires that have been designed for use with young people in North America are provided (see Figures 3.1 and 3.2). Some modifications are recommended to make them more appropriate for use with young people in the UK (see activity on p. 73).

Figure 3.1 The Physical Activity Questionnaire for Adolescents (PAQ-A)

Name: _____   Age: _____
Sex: M _____   F _____
Teacher: _____

We are trying to find out about your level of physical activity from the last 7 days (in the last week). This includes sports or dance that make you sweat or make your legs feel tired, or games that make you breathe hard, like tag, skipping, running, climbing and others.

Remember:

A) **There are no right and wrong answers – this is not a test.**
B) **Please answer all the questions as honestly and accurately as you can – this is very important.**

---

1. **PHYSICAL ACTIVITY IN YOUR SPARE TIME: Have you done any of the following activities in the past 7 days (last week)? If yes, how many times? (Mark only one circle per row).**

	No	1–2	3–4	5–6	7 times or more
Skipping	0	0	0	0	0
Rowing	0	0	0	0	0
In-line skating	0	0	0	0	0
Tag	0	0	0	0	0
Walking for exercise	0	0	0	0	0
Bicycling	0	0	0	0	0
Jogging or running	0	0	0	0	0
Aerobics	0	0	0	0	0
Swimming	0	0	0	0	0
Baseball, softball	0	0	0	0	0
Dance	0	0	0	0	0
Football	0	0	0	0	0
Badminton	0	0	0	0	0
Skateboarding	0	0	0	0	0
Soccer	0	0	0	0	0
Street hockey	0	0	0	0	0
Volleyball	0	0	0	0	0
Floor hockey	0	0	0	0	0
Basketball	0	0	0	0	0
Ice skating	0	0	0	0	0
Cross-country skiing	0	0	0	0	0
Ice hockey/ringette	0	0	0	0	0
Other	0	0	0	0	0

2. In the last 7 days, *during your physical education (PE) classes*, how often were you very active (playing hard, running, jumping, throwing)? (Check one only).

I don't do PE	0
Hardly ever	0
Sometimes	0
Quite often	0
Always	0

3. In the last 7 days, what did you normally do *at lunch* (besides eating lunch)? (Check one only).

Sat down (talking, reading, doing school work)	0
Stood around or walked around	0
Ran or played a little bit	0
Ran around or played quite a bit	0
Ran and played hard most of the time	0

4. In the last 7 days, on how many days *right after school*, did you do sports, dance, or play games in which you were very active? (Check one only).

none	0
1 time last week	0
2 or 3 times last week	0
4 times last week	0
5 times last week	0

5. In the last 7 days, on how many *evenings*, did you do sports, dance, or play games in which you were very active? (Check one only).

none	0
1 time last week	0
2 or 3 times last week	0
4 times last week	0
5 times last week	0

6. *On the last weekend*, how many times did you do sports, dance, or play games in which you were very active? (Check one only).

none	0
1 time	0
2–3 times	0
4–5 times	0
6 or more times	0

7. Which *one* of the following describes you best for the last 7 days? Read ALL FIVE statements before deciding on the *one* answer that describes you.

A) All or most of my free time was spent doing things involving little   0
   physical effort

B) I sometimes (1–2 times last week) did physical things in my free time 0

C) I quite often (3–4 times last week) did physical things in my free time 0

D) I often (5–6 times last week) did physical things in my free time   0

E) I very often (7 or more times last week) did physical things in my   0
   free time

8. Mark how often you did physical activity (like playing sports, games, doing dance, or any other physical activity) for each day last week.

	None	Little bit	Medium	Often	Very often
Monday	0	0	0	0	0
Tuesday	0	0	0	0	0
Wednesday	0	0	0	0	0
Thursday	0	0	0	0	0
Friday	0	0	0	0	0
Saturday	0	0	0	0	0
Sunday	0	0	0	0	0

9. Were you sick last week, or did anything prevent you from doing your normal physical activities? (Check one).

Yes   0
No   0
If yes, what prevented you?

Scoring

The eight items are each scored on a 5-point scale to give a summary total activity score. The PAQ-A composite is calculated as the mean of the eight items. Question 9 is not used in the calculation of the summary activity score.

Source: Kowalski, Crocker & Kowalski (1997). Reprinted
with permission.

The questionnaires include two types of format. The first involves a recall of activity over a representative period of time (e.g. a week, as in the PAQ-A (Physical Activity Questionnaire for Adolescents) (Kowalski, Crocker & Kowalski, 1997)), and the second (e.g. the Leisure Time Exercise Questionnaire (Godin & Shephard, 1985)), uses more general

Figure 3.2   The Leisure Time Exercise Questionnaire (LTEQ)

Name _____ Teacher _____ Class _____ Date _____

1) **Considering a 7-day period (a week), how many times on the average do you do the following kinds of exercise FOR MORE THAN 15 MINUTES during your free time? (write the appropriate number)**

TIMES PER WEEK

a) STRENUOUS EXERCISE
(HEART BEATS RAPIDLY)   _____
(i.e. running, jogging, hockey, football, squash,
basketball, cross country, skiing, judo, roller skating,
vigorous swimming, vigorous long distance bicycling)

b) MODERATE EXERCISE
(NOT EXHAUSTING)   _____
(i.e. fast walking, baseball, tennis, easy bicycling,
volleyball, badminton, easy swimming dancing)

c) MILD EXERCISE
(MINIMAL EFFORT)   _____
(i.e. yoga, archery, fishing from river bank,
bowling, golf, easy walking)

2) **Considering a 7-days period (a week), during your leisure-time, how often do you engage in any regular activity long enough to work up a sweat (or breathe hard)?**

Please circle your answer

OFTEN   **SOMETIMES**   **NEVER/RARELY**

SCORING

The first question is scored by multiplying the values by an intensity factor (3, 5 and 9 for mild, moderate and strenuous activity respectively) to yield a total index of physical activity for the week. The second question can be used as an additional measure of activity or as a check on the first question (e.g. children reporting a lot of activity in question 1 should indicate frequent sweating in question 2).

Source: Godin & Shephard (1985). Reprinted with permission.

questions about typical exercise behaviour. Alternatively, young people could be asked to keep physical activity diaries over a specified period or complete ROAs (Records of Achievement) or Pupil Profiles designed to include information on physical activity participation (Cale, 1998).

More recently, computer-based physical activity questionnaires have become increasingly popular and have advantages over 'paper and pencil assessments' (Welk & Wood, 2000). For example, ACTIVITY-GRAM is a computerized assessment available with the revised FITNESS-GRAM software (Cooper Institute for Aerobics Research, 1999) that has been designed for use within the curriculum. Default settings and prompts assist in completing the assessment, and the scoring and interpretation of the data are processed automatically. Further, the results provide personalized information and feedback (Welk & Wood, 2000). Computer-based assessments also promote and reinforce information technology skills.

Activity

Select one of the example physical activity questionnaires (Figure 3.1 or 3.2). For the chosen questionnaire, consider:

1 what modifications might need to be made to the form if it was to be administered to a group of 12-year-old British children;
2 the merits and drawbacks of the questionnaire;
3 what procedures might be followed in administering the questionnaire to ensure that the data collected were as accurate and reliable as possible.

Using the physical activity information

Having gathered information on young people's physical activity levels, it may be used in a variety of practical ways. Within a health care setting, Rice & Howell (2000) recommend that the evaluation of physical activity and physical fitness should be included in the complete assessment of young people. They note that, as well as assessing activity patterns, health care practitioners should counsel children and parents about adopting and maintaining regular physical activity. As highlighted earlier, within the educational and PE context, Cale (1998) and Welk & Wood (2000) suggest a number of uses for physical activity assessments which again are considered applicable to other practical contexts. For example:

1 To enhance instruction on physical activity concepts (e.g. the importance of physical activity, that moderate activity is good for health, what the constraints/barriers to participation are, how these can be overcome, etc.).
2 To facilitate goal-setting and self-monitoring of physical activity (e.g. using the information as the basis for setting realistic goals to increase or maintain physical activity levels).

3 To diagnose activity needs for individual exercise prescription
   (e.g. to establish whether a young person is meeting current physical
   activity recommendations and therefore what their activity needs are).
4 To promote young people's personal activity knowledge (e.g. about
   their current activity levels) and self-evaluation skills (e.g. to enable
   them to plan and make decisions about their physical activity).
5 To promote key skills through PE (e.g. problem-solving, improving
   own learning and performance, information technology) or cross-
   curricular links with other subjects (e.g. handling, presenting and
   interpreting data in mathematics).

References

ACSM (American College of Sports Medicine) (1988) Opinion statement on
  physical fitness in children and youth, *Medicine and Science in Sport and Exercise*,
  20(4), 422–3.

ACSM (American College of Sports Medicine) (2000) Exercise testing and
  prescription for children, the elderly, and pregnant women. In *ACSM's Guidelines
  for Exercise Testing and Prescription*, 6th edn. Philadelphia, PA: Lippincott
  Williams & Wilkins, 217–34.

American Alliance for Health, Physical Education, and Recreation (1976) *AAHPER
  Youth Test Manual*. Washington, DC: AAHPER.

Armstrong, N. (1987) A critique of fitness testing. In Biddle, S. (ed.), *Foundations
  of Health Related Fitness in Physical Education*. London: Ling Publishing House, 19–27.

Armstrong, N. (1989) Is fitness testing either valid or useful? *British Journal of
  Physical Education*, **20**, 66–7.

Armstrong, N. (1995) The assessment of health-related fitness in schools. In
  Darmody, M. & O'Donovan, G. (eds), *Physical Education at the Crossroads*.
  Limerick: PEAI, 44–8.

Armstrong, N. (1998) Young people's physical activity patterns as assessed by
  heart rate monitoring, *Journal of Sports Science*, **16**, S9–16.

Armstrong, N. & Biddle, S. (1992) Health-related physical activity in the
  national curriculum. In Armstrong, N. (ed.), *New Directions in Physical Education,
  Volume 2, Towards a National Curriculum*. Champaign, IL: Human Kinetics, 71–110.

Armstrong, N. & Van Mechelen, W. (1998) Are young people fit and active? In
  Biddle, S., Sallis, J. & Cavill, N. (eds), *Young and Active? Young People and Health-
  Enhancing Physical Activity – Evidence and Implications*. London: Health Education
  Authority, 69–97.

Armstrong, N. & Welsman, J. (1997) *Young People and Physical Activity*. Oxford:
  Oxford University Press.

Baranowski, T. (1988) Validity and reliability of self-report of physical activity:
  an information processing perspective, *Research Quarterly*, **59(4)**, 314–27.

Baranowski, T., Dworkin, R. J., Cieslik, C. J., et al. (1984) Reliability and validity of self-report of aerobic activity: Family Health Project 1,2, *Research Quarterly*, **55(4)**, 309–17.

Baranowski, T., & Simons-Morton, B. G. (1988) Children's physical activity and dietary assessments: measurement issues, *Journal of School Health*, **61**, 195–7.

Bar-Or, O. (1993) Importance of differences between children and adults for exercise testing and exercise prescription. In Skinner, J. S. (ed.), *Exercise Testing and Prescription for Special Cases*, 2nd edn. Lea Febiger, 57–74.

Bassett, D. R., Ainsworth, B. E. & Leggett, S. R. (1996) Accuracy of five electronic pedometers for measuring distance walked, *Medicine and Science in Sports and Exercise*, **28**, 1071–7.

Bassett, D. R., Ainsworth, B. E., Swartz, A. M., Strath, S. J., O'Brien, W. L. & King, G. A. (2000) Validity of four motion sensors in measuring moderate intensity physical activity, *Medicine and Science in Sports and Exercise*, **32**(supplement), S471–80.

Blimkie, C. J. R. & Macauley, D. (2000) Muscle strength. In Armstrong, N. & Van Mechelen, W. (eds), *Paediatric Exercise Science and Medicine*. Oxford: Oxford University Press, 23–36.

Boileau, R. A., Lohman, T. G., Slaughter, M. H., Horswill, G. A. & Stillman, R. J. (1986) Problems associated with determining body composition in maturing youngsters. In Brown, E. W. & Branta, C. F. (eds), *Competitive Sports for Children and Youth*. Champaign, IL: Human Kinetics, 3–16.

Bouchard, C. (1993) Heredity and health-related fitness, *President's Council on Physical Fitness and Sports Physical Activity and Fitness Research Digest*, **1(4)**, 1–8.

Bouchard, C., Dionne, F. T., Simoneau, J. & Boulay, M. (1992) Genetics of aerobic and anaerobic performances, *Exercise and Sport Sciences Reviews*, **20**, 27–58.

Brewer, J. & Davis, J. (1992; 2000) *Abdominal Curl Conditioning Test: A Progressive Sit-up Test*. Leeds: The National Coaching Foundation (now Sports Coach UK).

Brewer, J., Ramsbottom, R. & Williams, C. (1988) *Multistage Fitness Test*. Loughborough University and the National Coaching Foundation.

Brewer, J., Ramsbottom, R. & Williams, C. (2001) *Multistage Fitness Test*. Loughborough University and Sports Coach UK.

Cale, L. (1994) Self report measures of children's physical activity: recommendations for future development and a new alternative measure, *Health Education Journal*, **53**, 439–53.

Cale, L. (1998) Monitoring young people's physical activity, *The British Journal of Physical Education*, **29(2)**, 28–30.

Cale, L. & Harris, J. (1998) The benefits of health-related physical education and recommendations for implementation, *The Bulletin of Physical Education*, **34(1)**, 27–41.

Cale, L. & Harris, J. (2002) National fitness testing for children – issues, concerns and alternatives, *The British Journal of Teaching Physical Education*, **33(1)**, 32–34.

Caspersen, C. J., Powell, K. E. & Christenson, G. M. (1985) Physical activity, exercise and physical fitness: definitions and distinctions for health-related research, *Public Health Reports*, **100**, 126–30.

Claessens, A. L., Beunen, G. & Malina, R. M. (2000) Anthropometry, physique, body composition and maturity. In Armstrong, N. & Van Mechelen, W. (eds), *Paediatric Exercise Science and Medicine*. Oxford: Oxford University Press, 11–21.

Cooper, A. (2003) Objective measurement of physical activity. In McKenna, J. & Riddoch, C. (eds), *Perspectives on Health and Exercise*. Basingstoke: Palgrave Macmillan, 83–108.

Cooper Institute for Aerobics Research (1999) *FITNESSGRAM Test Administration Manual*, 2nd edn. Champaign, IL: Human Kinetics.

Corbin, C. B. (2002) Physical activity for everyone: what every physical educator should know about promoting lifelong physical activity, *Journal of Teaching in Physical Education*, **21**, 128–44.

Corbin, C. B. & Lindsey, R. (2002) *Fitness for Life*, 4th edn. Champaign, IL: Human Kinetics.

Cureton, K. J. (1994) Physical fitness and activity standards for youth. In Pate, R. R., & Hohn, R. C. (eds), *Health and Fitness Through Physical Education*. Champaign, IL: Human Kinetics, 129–36.

Cureton, K. J. & Warren, G., (1990) Criterion-referenced standards for youth health-related fitness tests: a tutorial, *Research Quarterly for Exercise and Sport*, **61**, 7–19.

Docherty, D (1996) Field tests and test batteries. In Docherty, D. (ed.), *Measurement in Pediatric Exercise Science*. Champaign, IL: Human Kinetics, 285–321.

Docherty, D. & Bell, R. (1990) Fitness testing: counterproductive to a healthy lifestyle? *CAHPER Journal*, **56(5)**, 4–8.

Durant, R. H., Baranowski, T., Davis, H. et al., (1993) Reliability and variability of heart rate monitoring in children, *Medicine and Science in Sports and Exercise*, **25(3)**, 389–95.

Emons, H. J. G., Groenenboom, D. C., Westerterp, K. R. & Saris, W. H. M. (1992) Comparison of heart rate monitoring combined with indirect calorimetry and the doubly labelled water ($^2H_2\,^{18}O$) method for the measurement of energy expenditure in children, *European Journal of Applied Physiology*, **65**, 99–103.

Eston, R. G., Rowlands, A. V. & Ingledew, D. K. (1998) Validity of heart rate, pedometry and accelerometry for predicting the energy cost of children's activities, *Journal of Applied Physiology*, **84(1)**, 362–71.

Eve, N. & Williams, D. (2000) Multistage fitness test in secondary schools – advice on safety, *Bulletin of Physical Education*, **36(2)**, 110–14.

Fox, K. & Biddle, S. (1986) Health related fitness testing in schools: introduction and problems of interpretation, *The Bulletin of Physical Education*, **22**, 54–64.

Freedson, P. S. (1991) Electronic motion sensors and heart rate as measures of physical activity in children, *Journal of School Health*, **61(5)**, 220–3.

Gibbons, R. J., Balady, G. J., Beasley, J. W. et al. (1997) ACC/AHA guidelines for exercise testing. A report of the American College of Cardiology/American Heart Association Task Force on practice guidelines (Committee on Exercise Testing), *Journal of the American College of Cardiology*, **30**, 260–315.

Godin, G. & Shephard, R. J. (1985) A simple method to assess exercise behaviour in the community, *Canadian Journal of Applied Sports Sciences*, **10(3)**, 141–6.

Harris, J. (1995) Physical education – a picture of health?, *The British Journal of Physical Education* **26(4)**, 25–32.

Harris, J. (2000) *Health-Related Exercise in the National Curriculum. Key Stages 1 to 4.* Leeds: Human Kinetics.

Harris, J. & Cale, L. (1997). How healthy is school PE? A review of the effectiveness of health-related physical education programmes in schools, *Health Education Journal*, **56**, 84–104.

Harris, J. & Elbourn, J. (1994) Measure for measure. Does activity and fitness monitoring have a place within physical education? *Sports Teacher*, **Autumn**, 11–15.

Harro, M. & Riddoch, C. (2000) Physical activity. In Armstrong, N. & Van Mechelen, W. (eds), *Paediatric Exercise Science and Medicine.* Oxford: Oxford University Press, 77–84.

Hopple, C. & Graham, G., (1995) What children think, feel and know about physical fitness testing, *Journal of Teaching in Physical Education*, **14(4)**, 408–17.

Janz, K. F., Neilsen, D. H., Cassady, S. L., Cook, J. S., Wu, Y.-T. & Hansen, J. R. (1993) Cross-validation of the Slaughter skinfold equations for children and adolescents, *Medicine and Science in Sports and Exercise*, **25**, 1070–976.

Kemper, H. C. G (1985) Growth, health and fitness of teenagers, *Medicine and Sport Science*, **20**, 1–202.

Kohl, H. W., Fulton, J. E. & Caspersen, C. J. (2000) Assessment of physical activity among children and adolescents: a review and synthesis, *Preventive Medicine*, **31**, S54–76.

Kowalski, K. C., Crocker, P. R. E. & Kowalski, N. P. (1997) Convergent validity of the physical activity questionnaire for adolescents, *Pediatric Exercise Science*, **9**, 342–52.

Livingstone, M. B. E., Coward, A. W., Prentice, A. M., Davies, P. S. W., Strain, J. J., McKenna, P. G., et al. (1992) Daily energy expenditure in free-living children: comparison of heart rate monitoring with the doubly labelled water ($^2H_2{}^{18}O$) method, *American Journal of Clinical Nutrition*, **56**, 343–52.

Lohman, T. G. (1989) Assessment of body composition in children, *Pediatric Exercise Science*, **1**, 19–30.

Lohman, T. G. (1992) *Advances in Body Composition Assessment.* Champaign, IL: Human Kinetics.

Lohman, T. G., Boileau, R. A. & Slaughter, M. H. (1984) Body composition in children and youth. In Boileau, R. A. (ed), *Advances in Pediatric Sports Science.* Champaign, IL: Human Kinetics, 229–57.

McKenzie, T. L. (1991) Observational measures of children's physical activity, *Journal of School Health*, **61(5)**, 224–7.

Melanson, E. L. & Freedson, P. S. (1996) Physical activity assessment: a review of methods, *Critical Reviews in Food Science and Nutrition*, **36**, 385–96.

O'Hara, N., Baranowski, T., Simons-Morton, B., Wilson, S. & Parcel, G. (1989) Validity of the observation of children's physical activity, *Research Quarterly for Exercise and Sport*, **60(1)**, 42–7.

Pangrazi, R. P. (2000) Promoting physical activity for youth, *The ACHPER Healthy Lifestyles Journal*, **47(2)**, 18–21.

Pangrazi, R. P. & Corbin, C. B. (1990) Age as a factor relating to physical fitness test performance, *Research Quarterly for Exercise and Sport*, **61(4)**, 410–14.

Pate, R. (1991) Health-related measures of children's physical fitness, *Journal of School Health*, **61**, 231–3.

Pate, R. R. (1988) The evolving definition of physical fitness, *Quest*, **40**, 174–9.

Pate, R. R. (1993) Physical activity assessment in children and adolescents, *Critical Reviews in Food Science and Nutrition*, **33(4–5)**, 321–6.

Pate, R. R. (1994) Fitness testing: current approaches and purposes in physical education. In Pate, R. R. & Hohn, R. C. (eds), *Health and Fitness Through Physical Education*. Champaign, IL: Human Kinetics, 119–27.

Pate, R. R., Ross, J. G., Baumgartner, T. E. & Sparks, R. E. (1987) The modified pull-up, *Journal of Physical Education and Recreation*, **58**, 71–3.

Pate, R. R., & Shephard, R. J. (1989) Characteristics of physical fitness in youth. In Gisolfi, C. V. & Lamb, D. R. (eds), *Perspectives in Exercise Science and Sports Medicine, Volume 2, Youth, Exercise and Sport*. Indianapolis, IN: Benchmark Press, 1–46.

PEA (Physical Education Association) (1988) Health related fitness testing and monitoring in schools. A position statement on behalf of the PEA by its fitness and health advisory committee, *British Journal of Physical Education*, **19(4/5)**, 194–5.

Perrin, D. H. (1993) *Isokinetic Exercise and Assessment*. Champaign, IL: Human Kinetics.

Puhl, J., Greaves, K., Hoyt, M. & Baranowski, T. (1990) Children's activity rating scale (CARS): description and calibration, *Research Quarterly for Exercise and Sport*, **61(1)**, 26–36.

Rice, M. H. & Howell, C. C. (2000) Measurement of physical activity, exercise, and physical fitness in children: issues and concerns, *Journal of Pediatric Nursing*, **15(3)**, 148–56.

Riddoch, C. J., Mahoney, C., Murphy, N., Cran, G. & Boreham, C. (1991) The physical activity patterns of Northern Irish schoolchildren ages 11–16 years, *Pediatric Exercise Science*, **3**, 300–9.

Ridley, K., Dollman, J. & Olds, T. (2001) Development and validation of a computer delivered physical activity questionnaire (CDPAQ) for children, *Pediatric Exercise Science*, **13**, 35–46.

Ross, J. G. (1989) Evaluating fitness and activity assessments from the National Children and Youth Fitness Studies I and II. In *Assessing Physical Fitness and Physical Activity in Population-Based Surveys*. Rockville, MD: US Department of Health and Human Services, Publication (PHS) DHSS, 89–1253.

Ross, J. G. & Gilbert, G. G. (1985) The national children and youth fitness study: a summary of findings, *Journal of Physical Education, Recreation and Dance*, **56**, 45–50.

Rowland, T. W. (1995) The horse is dead; let's dismount, *Pediatric Exercise Science*, **7**, 117–20.

Rowlands, A. V., Eston, R. G. & Ingledew, D. K. (1997) Measurement of physical activity in children with particular reference to the use of heart rate and pedometry, *Sports Medicine*, **24(4)**, 258–72.

Safrit, M. (1990) The validity and reliability of fitness tests for children: A review, *Pediatric Exercise Science*, **2**, 9–28.

Safrit, M. J., & Looney, M. A. (1992) Should the punishment fit the crime? A measurement dilemma, *Research Quarterly for Exercise and Sport*, **62**, 124–7.

Sallis, J. F. (1991) Self-report measures of children's physical activity, *Journal of School Health*, **61(5)**, 215–19.

Sallis, J. F., Buono, M. J., Roby, J. et al. (1990) The Caltrac accelerometer as a physical activity monitor for school-age children, *Medicine and Science in Sports and Exercise*, **22(5)**, 698–703.

Saris, W. H. M. (1985) The assessment and evaluation of daily physical activity in children: a review, *Acta Paediatrica Scandinavica*, **318**, 37–48.

Saris, W. H. M. (1986) Habitual physical activity in children: methodology and findings in health and disease, *Medicine and Science in Sports and Exercise*, **18(3)**, 253–63.

Schoeller, D. A. (1983) Energy expenditure from doubly labeled water: some fundamental considerations in humans, *American Journal of Clinical Nutrition*, **38**, 999–1005.

Seefeldt, V. & Vogel, P. (1989) Physical fitness testing of children: a 30-year history of misguided efforts, *Pediatric Exercise Science*, **1**, 295–302.

Sirard, J. R. & Pate, R. R. (2001) Physical activity assessment in children and adolescents, *Sports Medicine*, **31(6)**, 439–54.

Skinner, J. (1993) *Exercise Testing and Exercise Prescription for Special Cases*, 2nd edn. Philadelphia: Lea & Febiger.

Slaughter, M. H., Lohman, T. G., Boileau, R. A., Horswill, C. A., Stillman, R. J., VanLoan, M. D. et al. (1988) Skinfold equations for examination of body fatness in children and youth, *Human Biology*, **60**, 709–23.

Tomassoni, T. L. (1996) Introduction: the role of exercise in the diagnosis and management of chronic disease in children and youth, *Medicine and Science in Sports and Exercise*, **28**, 403–5.

Treiber, F. A., Musante, L., Hartdagan, S., Davis, H., Levy, M. & Strong, W. B. (1989) Validation of a heart rate monitor with children in laboratory and field settings, *Medicine and Science in Sports and Exercise*, **21**, 338–42.

Verschuur, R. & Kemper, H. C. G. (1985) Habitual physical activity in Dutch teenagers measured by heart rate. In Binkhorst, R. A., Kemper, H. C. G., & Saris, W. H. M (eds), *Children and Exercise XI*. Champaign, IL: Human Kinetics, 194–202.

Wareham, N. J. & Rennie, K. L. (1998) The assessment of physical activity in individuals and populations: why try to be more precise about how physical activity is assessed? *International Journal of Obesity*, **22**(supplement 2), S30–38.

Welk, G. J., Corbin, C. B. & Dale, D. (2000) Measurement issues in the assessment of physical activity in children, *Research Quarterly for Exercise and Sport*, **71**(2), 59–73.

Welk, G. J. & Wood, K. (2000) Physical activity assessments in physical education. A practical review of instruments and their use in the curriculum, *Journal of Physical Education, Recreation, and Dance*, **71**(1), 30–40.

Whitehead, J. R., Pemberton, C. L. & Corbin, C. B. (1990) Perspectives on the physical fitness testing of children: the case for a realistic educational approach, *Pediatric Exercise Science*, **2**, 111–23.

4

The Determinants of Physical Activity and Inactivity in Young People

Trish Gorely

As outlined in Chapter 2, there are potentially important health outcomes for young people from regular participation in physical activity. Despite this, and whilst children and adolescents are generally considered to be the most active population group with many demonstrating good participation levels (e.g. Department of Health and Human Services & Centers for Disease Control and Prevention, 1996; WHO, 2000) and meeting physical activity guidelines (e.g. Armstrong & Van Mechelen, 1998; Joint Health Surveys Unit, 1998; Gregory & Lowe, 2000), it remains a concern that still a sizeable number are inactive and lead sedentary lifestyles (Joint Health Surveys Unit, 1998; Gregory & Lowe, 2000) (see Chapter 2). Further, the polarization of activity levels evident in today's youth (Cavill, 2001) begs the question why some young people are active and others are not. In order to answer this question, there is clearly a need to examine the determinants of physical activity in this age group (Sallis, Prochaska & Taylor, 2000).

Another way of addressing the issue of young people's activity levels is to examine what it is that young people do when they are being 'inactive' (Marshall et al., 2002), and there have been recent calls to study sedentary behaviour as a concept distinct from physical activity (Owen et al., 2000). Many young people find sedentary behaviours more reinforcing than physically active alternatives and appear more likely to choose sedentary activities even when physically active alternatives are freely available (Epstein et al., 1991; Vara & Epstein, 1993). This chapter also discusses the determinants of some of the most prevalent sedentary behaviours. By identifying consistent determinants of these behaviours, more effective interventions to reduce them may be possible, resulting in increases in physical activity levels. For example, there is evidence that reducing sedentary behaviour without specifically targeting active behaviours can increase levels of physical activity (Epstein & Roemmich, 2001).

Discussion point   What factors influenced your participation in physical activity when you were young?

What factors influence your participation now? Discuss any similarities and differences.

The term determinants, as it has generally been employed in the literature, refers to reproducible but not necessarily causal associations between a behaviour (physical activity) and some factor such as gender or self-confidence (Buckworth & Dishman, 2002). Because of the lack of a cause-and-effect relationship there has been a call recently to use the more technically correct term of 'correlates' to describe these associations (Bauman et al., 2002). Knowing the characteristics of those who are active and those who are not is helpful in intervention design (Sallis, Prochaska & Taylor, 2000). Unmodifiable correlates (e.g. age, gender) can be used to identify target groups for interventions. Modifiable correlates (e.g. self-efficacy) are factors that can be targeted for change during the intervention, thus making change in physical activity behaviour more likely (Baranowski, Anderson, & Carmack, 1998).

An ecological approach to physical activity

The majority of early research on the correlates of physical activity focused on individually oriented psychological and social variables which have subsequently been shown to explain only a small amount of variance (Giles-Corti & Donovan, 2002; Sallis, Kraft, & Linton, 2002). This focus has been criticized for ignoring how the environment may be facilitating or inhibiting physical activity behaviour (Stokols, 1992; Giles-Corti & Donovan, 2002). Recognition of the limitations of an individualistic focus has led to the development of ecological approaches to physical activity (Sallis & Owen, 1997; Sallis, Bauman, & Pratt, 1998; Spence & Lee, 2003). Ecological approaches have, at their core, the notion that behaviour, in this case physical activity, is influenced by multiple facets of the intrapersonal, interpersonal and physical, and policy and legislative environments (see Figure 4.1). This consideration of multiple levels of influence further distinguishes ecological models from other theoretical perspectives. This chapter uses an ecological perspective to structure the discussion of correlates and how this information can then be applied in practice.

In biology, ecology is the study of the interrelations between organisms and their environments (Stokols, 1992). An ecological perspective in the behavioural sciences focuses on people's interactions and relationships with their physical and social environment (Sallis & Owen, 2002). It is suggested that individuals adapt their behaviour in response to changes in the physical and social environment (Spence & Lee, 2003). The ecological approach provides a general framework for explaining behaviour, rather

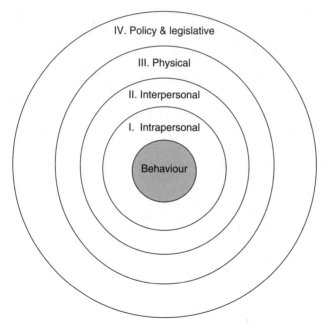

Figure 4.1 Levels of influence on behaviour from an ecological perspective

than a series of specific constructs or variables. Because of this generality, other theories and models that have been used in the exercise domain (e.g. Social Cognitive Theory, Theory of Planned Behaviour, (see Chapter 6)) can be incorporated to increase specificity (Smedley & Syme, 2000).

According to Stokols (1992), there are four assumptions underpinning ecological approaches to understanding health behaviours. First, health behaviours are influenced by multiple facets of the physical and social environments, along with a variety of personal factors (e.g. psychological characteristics and behavioural patterns). Secondly, the environments themselves are multidimensional and complex. For example, environments have social and physical components, there are differences between the actual environment and people's perceptions of the environment, and environments can be described in terms of discrete attributes (e.g. lighting, group size) or as a composite of these. Thirdly, the individual–environment interaction can be described at various levels of aggregation (individuals, families, workplaces, communities, countries). Finally, ecological approaches imply reciprocal causation in person–environment interactions, with the behaviour both influencing and being influenced by the environment. There is also an acknowledgement that determinants interact across environments (e.g. exercise facilities may be influenced by the socio-economic status of an area).

The actual levels of influence within this approach have been conceptualized in a variety of ways. Bronfenbrenner (1979) suggested there were micro-, meso-, exo-, and macrosystem levels of influence. The microsystem level involves face-to-face influences in specific settings, such as in the family or at school, and the mesosystem level involves interrelations between the various settings (microsystems) in which the person is involved (e.g. church, family and school). The exosystem is the larger social system that the person is part of, whereas the macrosystem refers to cultural beliefs and values. Each of these levels is proposed to facilitate or constrain certain behaviours, but the most proximal levels (i.e. microsystem and mesosystem) are thought to have the most direct and explicit influence. Spence & Lee (2003) have recently built on this model to develop a comprehensive ecological model for physical activity. Another perspective in levels of influence was proposed by McLeroy et al. (1988), who suggested five levels of behavioural determinants:

1 intrapersonal (e.g. psychological and biological variables and developmental history);
2 interpersonal (e.g. family, peers and co-workers);

3 institutional (e.g. schools and worksites);
4 community (e.g. relationships between organizations and institutions within a local area);
5 public policy (e.g. laws and policies of local and national governments).

The advantage of dividing the environment into different levels of influence is that it forces attention on the potential for greater understanding and improved intervention at each level. Although McLeroy et al. (1988) do not specifically include physical environments, these are now recognized as central components of the ecological approach (Sallis, Bauman & Pratt, 1998), giving rise to the notion of a 'behaviour setting'. Behaviour settings are the physical and social context in which behaviour occurs (Barker, 1968). Some settings promote physical activity (e.g. parks, playgrounds, health clubs) and others discourage or prohibit physical activity (e.g. classrooms, offices). Further, the influence of the physical environment can be passive or active (Giles-Corti & Donovan, 2002). Passive influences are through the effects of urban environment, building design, or technological advances in domestic appliances which influence incidental exercise (e.g. the stairs in many buildings are hard to find, poorly lit and sometimes locked, thus discouraging stair use, while elevators and escalators are well lit and central, and therefore readily accessible). Active effects are those that occur through the provision of opportunities to participate in physical activity in accessible, safe, convenient and appealing environments (e.g. the provision of a well-lit, widespread network of footpaths or cycle lanes).

Ecological approaches provide a framework for understanding the complex interplay between the many personal and environmental influences on behaviour. Because of the multiple-level perspective, eco-logical approaches are inherently complex. However, the broader nature of these approaches may ultimately lead to more successful interventions by encouraging efforts at more than the level of the individual (Giles-Corti & Donovan, 2002).

Theories/models used to study correlates of physical activity

An ecological approach does not exclude models and theories that have been used to focus on individual social and psychological correlates of physical activity (see Chapter 6 for an overview of models and approaches to physical activity promotion). Rather, it draws on these theories, where appropriate, to add specificity to the explanation of how or why a particular factor may influence behaviour. The common models that have been employed in this field are Social Cognitive Theory (Bandura, 1986), the Theory of Reasoned Action and the Theory of Planned Behaviour (Ajzen, 1991; Fishbein & Ajzen, 1975) (see Chapter 6). Alongside theory-driven studies, there have been a number of atheoretical examinations of correlates or studies employing combinations of variables drawn from several theories (Sallis & Owen, 1999). Despite the variability in the application of theories and models, an understanding of the basic tenets of the main theories employed is useful when interpreting the general findings of correlates research, and may provide an explanation of how or why a particular correlate affects behaviour. No one theory, however, is likely to explain the complex of influences on physical activity behaviour.

Correlates of physical activity in young people

The most comprehensive and systematic review of the correlates of physical activity in young people is provided by Sallis, Prochaska & Taylor (2000), and the main findings of this review (see Table 4.1 for a summary) are used to identify key correlates of young people's physical activity here. Although systematically reviewing all papers published in a 28-year period (1970–98), the review by Sallis and colleagues focused on the correlates of overall physical activity and excluded studies with a primary focus on sports participation. This is considered a potential limitation of the work, given the centrality of sports participation to children's physical activity (Vilhjalmsson & Kristjansdottir, 2003). In line with the review, a distinction is made between children (less than 13 years of age) and adolescents (13–18 years) where possible.

While reading this section it is important to bear in mind that the study of correlates in young people is complicated by the rapid psychological, physical and social developmental changes that are occurring in this age group (Sallis & Owen, 1999). The effects of these changes are not well understood, and in the case of some variables (e.g. psychological correlates), the developmental effects may be difficult or impossible to elucidate because the young person may lack the cognitive ability to self-report on these variables (Sallis & Owen, 1999; Sallis, Prochaska & Taylor, 2000).

Intrapersonal factors

For demographic and biological variables, the results from Sallis, Prochaska & Taylor (2000) suggest that even at a young age males are more

Table 4.1 Summary of the results from a review of correlates of physical activity of children and adolescents

Determinant variable	Children 4–12 yrs		Adolescents 13–18 yrs	
	Association	k	Association	k
Intrapersonal influences				
Demographic and biological				
Age	??	19	—	27
Ethnicity (EuroAm)	??	11	++	14
Sex (male)	++	31	++	28
Socioeconomic status	00	13	00	9
Single parent status	0	4		
Body mass index	??	31	00	21
Parent overweight/obesity	+	5		
Psychological/cognitive factors				
Self-esteem	00	6	00	9
Perceived competence	??	7	+	3
Self-efficacy	??	9	??	13
Body image	00	4	??	7
Attitudes, outcome expectations	??	14	??	7
Sweat attitudes	00	4		
After school activity attitudes	00	4		
Dislikes PE	00	5	??	9
PA intention	+	5	++	8
PA preference	+	5		
Perceived benefits	00	7	??	29
General barriers	—	3	00	15
Achievement orientation			++	6

Table 4.1 (Continued)

Determinant variable	Children 4–12 yrs		Adolescents 13–18 yrs	
	Association	k	Association	k
Talks loudly			0	0
External locus of control			00	4
Self-motivation			0	3
Enjoy exercise			00	5
Stress			00	7
Depression			–	4
Knowledge of exercise/health			??	7
Behavioural attributes and skills				
Cigarette use	0	3	??	15
Alcohol use	0	3	00	13
Healthy diet	+	3	00	16
Caloric intake	0	3		
Previous PA	‡+	6	‡+	12
Sedentary time	??	15	00	12
Sedentary after school			–	3
Sedentary on weekend			–	3
Sensation seeking			+	3
Fighting			00	4
Chewing tobacco			0	3
Meal regularity			?	4
Community sports			‡+	7
On school sports teams			0	3

Social and cultural factors				
Parent PA	??	29	00	27
Parent PA participation with youth	??	10		
Parent benefits of PA	0	3		
Parent barriers to PA	0	3		
Parental encouragement, persuasion	00	13	+	3
Parent transport child	00	8		
Parent pays PA fees	0	4		
Subjective norms	0	3	??	11
Peer influence/modelling	0	3	00	5
Sibling PA			‡	4
Direct parental help in PA			+	4
Teacher support or modelling			00	6
Support from significant others			‡	4
Support from peers			?	5
Coach support/modelling			00	6
Physical environment factors				
Access to facilities/programmes	+	4		
Parent provides transportation to PA	0	4		
Season (summer/spring)	?	4		
Milieu (rural)	?	4		

Table 4.1 (Continued)

Determinant variable	Children 4–12 yrs		Adolescents 13–18 yrs	
	Association	k	Association	k
Neighbourhood safety	00	4		
Time outdoors	+	3		
Equipment/supplies available			00	8
Opportunities to exercise			+	3
Sports media influence			0	3

Notes: k = number of independent samples in which this variable has been studied; EuroAm, European American; PA, physical activity; PE, physical education; −, negative association; +, positive association; 0, no association; ?, indeterminate/inconsistent association; Double codes (e.g. −, ++, 00) were used when four or more studies supported an association, no association; ?? indicates a variable that has been frequently studied with considerable lack of consistency in the findings.

Source: Sallis, Prochaska & Taylor (2000). Reprinted with permission.

active than females. Inconsistent findings were found for age, ethnicity and body mass index and there was no relationship between physical activity and body weight/fatness or socio-economic status (SES) in this age group. For adolescents, males are more active than females, as are non-Hispanic whites compared to all other ethnic groups. During adolescence there is a decrease in physical activity participation with increasing age. However, and as acknowledged in Chapter 2, there has been some debate surrounding this age-related decline recently, with some reporting the decline to be more pronounced in girls, and others arguing the opposite (see Sallis, 2000). This may be due to greater initial levels of activity in boys, although the inconsistency of conclusions may be the result of the time points studied. Also, some confounding between demographic correlates is possible; for example, the ethnicity results may be confounded by SES (Sallis, Prochaska & Taylor, 2000).

Few psychological variables have been comprehensively studied in children and adolescents, and none of the psychological theories described earlier have been extensively applied in this age group. Nonetheless, some of the components within these theories have received support. For example, in children there is some evidence that physical activity is associated with fewer perceived barriers, intentions to be active, and preferences for physical activity. However, inconsistent relationships were found for perceived competence, self-efficacy and attitudes/outcome expectations. For adolescents, achievement orientation,[1] perceived competence, and intention to be active were positively associated, and depression negatively associated, with physical activity. Self-efficacy, body image, attitudes/outcome expectations, liking of physical education, benefits of physical activity and knowledge of exercise/health were all inconsistently related to physical activity. The inconsistent finding for self-efficacy is particularly surprising given its centrality to adults' participation (McAuley & Mihalko, 1998) and to the psychological models used to explain physical activity behaviour. Sallis, Prochaska & Taylor (2000) found no association between physical activity and general barriers and enjoyment. This is in contrast to the qualitative work of

---

[1] Achievement orientation relates to how individuals define sucess. A task goal orientation focuses on comparing performance with personal standards and previous performance. An ego orientation focuses on comparing performance with others and winning.

Mulvihill, Rivers & Aggleton (2000) who found many barriers to emerge during the transition from primary to secondary school. Greater embarrassment and self-consciousness of their bodies, especially for girls, and perceived time pressure from homework were reported as barriers to physical activity by the young people. In contrast, the young people spoke of being motivated by feelings of wellbeing, enjoyment and possible weight control.

Despite the inconsistent findings for many psychological variables, it is probably too early to discount these factors, as methodological inconsistencies and measurement issues might account for a substantial portion of the variability in findings. As demonstrated by the work of Mulvihill, Rivers & Aggleton, (2000), qualitative approaches may offer further insight into psychological influences on physical activity participation.

Sallis, Prochaska & Taylor (2000) identified few studies that have examined behavioural variables in young people and, within these, only a small number of consistent associations were found. For children, healthy diet and previous physical activity were positively associated with activity. For adolescents, sensation-seeking, previous activity and participation in community sports showed positive relationships with physical activity. No consistent association was found between physical activity and sedentary behaviours in children (e.g. TV viewing), but in adolescents there was a negative relationship between physical activity and time in sedentary pursuits after school and at weekends.

Interpersonal factors

In contrast to narrative reviews (e.g. Wold & Hendry, 1998; Sallis & Owen, 1999), the semi-quantitative review by Sallis, Prochaska & Taylor (2000) found no social variables to be clearly associated with physical activity in children. Inconsistent findings were evident for the association between child physical activity levels and parent physical activity levels, or the parent participating with the child. No relationship was found between child physical activity levels and parental encouragement to participate, parental support for participation in the form of transport, or subjective norm or peer influence. In adolescence, parental support, support from significant others and sibling physical activity were positively associated with activity (Sallis, Prochaska & Taylor, 2000) but other social factors (e.g. peer modelling, perceived peer support) were not.

Apart from parental activity/modelling, few of the social variables have been extensively studied or consistently measured, meaning that it is also probably too early to discount their influence on both childhood and adolescent physical activity. It is possible that parental factors may have an indirect effect on participation through influences on perceived competence (McElroy, 2002). Wold & Hendry (1998) and Mulvihill, Rivers & Aggleton (2000) suggest that some peer influence is likely through a link with friendship patterns.

Prochaska, Rodgers & Sallis (2002) reported that, in adolescents, peer support was a stronger predictor of self-reported physical activity than parental support. However, neither peer or parental support was related to directly monitored physical activity. A possible explanation for this discrepancy lies in the nature of activity being measured by each method (see Chapter 3 for an overview of physical activity monitoring methods). Self-report measures typically focus on intentional physical activity and sports, whereas direct measures, such as accelerometry, record incidental physical activity throughout the day. These latter, more global and incidental activity levels may be less related to social support (Prochaska, Rodgers & Sallis, 2002). More research, using a combination of physical activity assessment methods is required to explore the influence of social variables and the social environment on youth physical activity.

Physical environment factors

Limited attention has been afforded to the influence of physical environmental factors on young people's physical activity. Despite this, consistent associations were reported by Sallis, Prochaska & Taylor (2000) for both children and adolescents. In children, access to facilities and programmes and time spent outside were both associated with greater physical activity. In adolescents, the broad construct of 'opportunities to exercise' was associated with greater activity. This may be a particularly important finding as continuing changes in the physical environment may further limit physical activity opportunities. For example, changes in urban design that encourage car use may limit opportunities for active travel (Frank & Engelke, 2002; Saelens, Sallis, & Frank, 2003). Greater attention needs to be paid to the influence of the physical environment on young people's physical activity participation.

Activity

Using the ecological model (see Figure 4.1), categorize the factors that you identified in the earlier discussion point into the appropriate levels of influence (I–IV). Which level(s) has/have had the most influence on your physical activity participation? Which has/have had the least influence? On reflection, do you consider any additional factors to be important?

Correlates of sedentary behaviours in young people

Understanding factors that influence participation in sedentary pursuits is important as young people can choose between a number of leisure activities, the majority of which are sedentary in nature – further, they seem to prefer these sedentary activities (Epstein et al., 1991; Vara & Epstein, 1993). In an effort to increase physical activity it would seem logical to try to understand the appeal and attraction of these sedentary pursuits.

Discussion point   In your view, can and should physical activity compete with sedentary activities in young people? What are the implications of young people's participation in sedentary activities for physical activity promotion?

Unfortunately, little is known about the aetiology of habitual sedentariness in young people or about the correlates of individual sedentary behaviours. One reason for this is that sedentary behaviour has seldom been explicitly assessed, with sedentariness typically being defined as 'activity absence'. That is, the physical activity level of participants has been assessed and those not reaching a certain criterion have been labelled as 'inactive' or 'sedentary'. While this gives an indication of levels of inactivity in the population, it tells us nothing about what these 'inactive' people are actually doing. Further, where sedentary behaviour has been measured more explicitly, inactivity has usually been based on levels of a single marker such as TV viewing. Use of single behaviours, however, may give an inaccurate assessment of inactivity levels because young people can find many ways of being inactive. For example, Marshall et al. (2002) used cluster analysis to investigate the interaction between physical activity and patterns of sedentary behaviour in a large sample of adolescents (11–16 years). They found three clusters for both boys ('techno-actives', 'non-socialising actives' and 'uninvolved inactives') and girls ('socialising actives', 'non-socialising actives' and 'uninvolved inactives'). The 40 per cent of boys in the 'techno-active' cluster were involved in higher than average TV and video game use but also in above-average physical activity. Thus, studying multiple behaviours concurrently is important to facilitate a more complete understanding of youth sedentariness and patterns of sedentary behaviour (Marshall et al., 2002).

As noted earlier, a few studies have examined the correlates of sedentary behaviours in youth, but most have focused on TV viewing. It has already been reported that Sallis, Prochaska & Taylor (2000) found inconsistent relationships between time spent on TV and video games and physical activity in children, and no relationship in adolescents. More recently, Schmitz et al. (2002) studied the psychosocial correlates of sedentary leisure habits in young adolescents (mean age 12.8 years) as part of the Teens Eating for Energy and Nutrition at School Study. A sedentary-leisure-habits score was calculated from self-reported TV viewing and video-game playing on weekdays and at weekends. For boys, sedentary leisure habits were positively associated with ethnicity (African-American) and depressive symptomology, and negatively associated with SES, spirituality, future expectations and aspirations for college. For girls, a positive relationship was found for ethnicity (African-American) and depressive symptomology, and a negative relationship was found between sedentary leisure habits and age, parent education, value of health, appearance and achievement scale, the authoritative mother scale and perceived academic rank. These findings suggest that demographic variables are the most robust predictors of sedentary leisure habits. This also supports the work of Gordon-Larsen, McMurray & Popkin (2000) who concluded that physical activity and inactivity were associated with different determinants, with physical activity being associated most strongly with environmental factors, and inactivity with socio-demographic factors. These conclusions must be treated with caution, however, as the systematic study of the correlates of inactivity in young people is still in its infancy and their importance lies mostly in identifying that the correlates of sedentary behaviour are likely to be different from those for physical activity. More attention needs to be given to this area of research.

Implications for physical activity interventions in young people

Understanding the correlates of physical activity and sedentary behaviour in young people is important for the development of effective physical activity interventions. The existence of unmodifiable correlates highlights that young people as a group are not homogenous, and any interventions should be differentiated on the basis of these correlates

(HEA, 1998). For example, the consistent findings for age, sex and ethnic differences suggest at least three target groups of individuals at risk for inactive lifestyles. Modifiable correlates provide direction on intervention content. If a correlate such as self-efficacy is a true determinant of physical activity then an intervention that successfully increases self-efficacy should also result in an increase in physical activity. This order is important – interventions based on modifiable determinants should primarily focus on changing the determinant that controls the behaviour and not the behaviour itself (Sallis & Owen, 1999). The review by Sallis, Prochaska & Taylor (2000) identified different correlates for children and adolescents, suggesting that different intervention strategies based around these age-specific correlates are required (Morrow, Jackson, & Payne, 1999).

Consistent correlates of physical activity have been identified in most domains proposed within an ecological approach. The study of correlates of sedentary behaviour is still too young to be in this position, but it is likely that, with more systematic study, correlates will be identified at each level. From an ecological perspective, and as Chapter 10 also suggests, interventions are likely to be most successful when they target changes in modifiable correlates across these multiple levels of influence (intrapersonal, interpersonal, physical environmental and policy) (Sallis, Bauman and Pratt, 1998). At the same time, there is a need for consistent interventions and messages across the multiple behaviour settings in which people engage (Resnicow, Robinson, & Frank, 1996; Sallis, Bauman and Pratt, 1998). For example, at the microsystem level of a school, it is likely that interventions will be most effective when they are integrated across a number of classes, deliver a unified message, and are supported by all levels of school administration (Wechsler et al., 2000) (see the notion of the 'Active School' in Chapter 7). However, it is unrealistic to expect schools to be able to facilitate major changes without the support of families and communities (i.e. the mesosystem) (Wechsler et al., 2000). Young people spend only some of their time in school and outside of school hours they may encounter powerful alternative messages to those they hear in school. From an ecological perspective, environmental interventions should be in place before educational interventions are undertaken (Sallis, Bauman and Pratt, 1998). That is, efforts should be made to provide an appropriate environment in which people can be active before targeting the behaviour. Finally, the combination of educational and environmental interventions varies depending on the behaviour setting (Sallis, Bauman and Pratt, 1998). Where interventions are being conducted in settings that encourage physical activity (e.g. school playgrounds), then educational and environmental strategies can be given equal emphasis. However, if the setting means physical activity is inappropriate, then educational strategies should be the prime emphasis.

As acknowledged later in the book (see Chapters 7 and 10), while the role of the school environment in influencing behaviour has been recognized, aside from changes to the PE curriculum (Stone et al., 1998), the effects of other school environment influences on physical activity have not been studied extensively (Wechsler et al., 2000). Wechsler et al. (2000) reviewed research examining four potentially influential school environment factors for physical activity: break periods, intramural sports and physical activity programmes, facilities that support physical activity, and psychosocial support for physical activity. These authors demonstrated that limited data on the contribution of these factors to the physical activity levels of young people are available and, while a logical argument can be made for their potential influence, research investigating how and in what circumstances these environmental factors operate is required.

Most interventions in the past have focused exclusively on increasing physical activity, but there is now evidence that interventions focused on reducing sedentary time may have positive effects on health outcomes. For example, in a randomized controlled school-based trial, Robinson (1999) showed that an intervention designed to decrease TV, videotape and video game use resulted in relatively smaller developmental gains in body mass index, triceps skinfold thickness, waist circumference and waist-to-hip ratio. Epstein and colleagues (Epstein, Saelens & O'Brien, 1995; Epstein et al., 1997) showed that reinforcing children for being less sedentary resulted in similar changes in physical activity levels compared to reinforcing children for being more active. Based on these findings, a joint approach, focused on increasing physical activity and decreasing sedentary behaviours, may have the greatest effect on overall physical activity behaviour change and health outcomes. Further, reducing sedentary behaviours in young people may be especially important as there is evidence that physical inactivity tracks better than physical activity from childhood to adolescence (Pate et al., 1999; Janz, Dawson, & Mahoney, 2000) and from adolescence to early adulthood (Raitakari et al., 1994; Malina, 1996).

Schmitz et al. (2002) examined the psychosocial correlates of physical activity and sedentary leisure habits within the same group of adolescents. They identified some common predictors of sedentary leisure behaviour and physical activity in girls but not in boys. For example, girls having an authoritative mother, placing higher value on health, appearance and achievement, and having a higher perceived academic rank, were associated with higher physical activity and lower sedentary behaviour. According to Schmitz et al., the existence of some common correlates may make it easier to intervene on both active and sedentary behaviours in the same intervention. Alternatively, factors influencing more than one behaviour may prove to be more difficult to change than factors associated with a single outcome.

Conclusions

Previous efforts to increase physical activity levels in young people have almost exclusively focused on physical activity behaviour but there is now evidence that intervention attention on decreasing sedentary behaviours may also result in increases in physical activity levels. The identification of consistent correlates of physical activity and sedentary behaviour is therefore considered important for the development of effective interventions. Consistent correlates have been identified in both children and adolescents for physical activity. However, the design of much of this work does not allow causality to be established and there is a need to conduct such work. Less is known about the correlates of sedentary behaviour as these have seldom been explicitly studied. The finding of consistent correlates of physical activity in most domains proposed within an ecological approach suggests that interventions will be most effective when they target multiple levels of influence.

Acknowledgements

The author would like to thank Professor Stuart Biddle and Dr Simon Marshall for their support in writing this chapter.

References

Ajzen, I. (1991) The theory of planned behavior, *Organizational Behavior and Human Decision Processes*, **50**, 179–211.

Armstrong, N. & Van Mechelen, W. (1998) Are young people fit and active? In Biddle, S., Sallis, J. & Cavill, N. (eds), *Young and Active? Young People and Health-Enhancing Physical Activity – Evidence and Implications*. London: Health Education Authority, 69–97.

Bandura, A. (1986) *Social Foundations of Thought and Action.* Englewood Cliffs, NJ: Prentice-Hall.

Baranowski, T., Anderson, C. & Carmack, C. (1998) Mediating frameworks in physical activity interventions: How are we doing? How might we do better? *American Journal of Preventive Medicine,* **15**, 266–97.

Barker, R. (1968) *Ecological Psychology: Concepts and Methods for Studying the Environment of Human Behavior.* Stanford, CA: Stanford University Press.

Bauman, A., Sallis, J., Dzewaltowski, D. & Owen, N. (2002) Toward a better understanding of the influences on physical activity: The role of determinants, correlates, causal variables, mediators, moderators, and confounders, *American Journal of Preventive Medicine,* **23(2S)**, 5–14.

Bronfenbrenner, U. (1979) *The Ecology of Human Development.* Cambridge, MA: Harvard University Press.

Buckworth, J. & Dishman, R. (2002) *Exercise Psychology.* Champaign, IL: Human Kinetics.

Cavill, N. (2001) Children and Young People – The Importance of Physical Activity. A paper published in the context of the European Heart Health Initiative. Brussels: European Heart Network.

Department of Health and Human Services & Centers for Disease Control and Prevention (1996) *Physical Activity and Health: A Report of the Surgeon General.* Atlanta, GA: Department of Health and Human Services & Center for Disease Control and Prevention.

Epstein, L. H. & Roemmich, J. N. (2001) Reducing sedentary behaviour: role in modifying physical activity, *Exercise and Sport Sciences Reviews,* **29**, 103–8.

Epstein, L. H., Saelens, B. E., Myers, M. D. & Vito, D. (1997) Effects of decreasing sedentary behaviors on activity choice in obese children, *Health Psychology,* **16(2)**, 107–13.

Epstein, L. H., Saelens, B. E. & O'Brien, J. G. (1995) Effects of reinforcing increases in active behavior versus decreases in sedentary behavior for obese children, *International Journal of Behavioral Medicine,* **2(1)**, 41–50.

Epstein, L. H., Smith, J. A., Vara, L. S. & Rodefer, J. S. (1991) Behavioral economic analysis of activity choice in obese children, *Health Psychology,* **10**, 311–16.

Fishbein, M. & Ajzen, I. (1975) *Belief, Attitude, Intention, and Behavior: An Introduction to Theory and Research.* Reading, MA: Addison-Wesley.

Frank, L. & Engelke, P. (2002) How land use and transportation systems impact public health: a literature review of the relationship between physical activity and built form. Available: http://www.cdc.gov/nccdphp/dnpa/pdf/aces-workingpaper1.pdf [18/07/2003].

Giles-Corti, B. & Donovan, R. J. (2002) The relative influence of individual, social and physical environment determinants of physical activity, *Social Science and Medicine,* **54**, 1793–812.

Gordon-Larsen, P., McMurray, R. G. & Popkin, B. M. (2000) Determinants of adolescent physical activity and inactivity patterns, *Pediatrics,* **105**, 1–8.

Gregory, J. & Lowe, S. (2000) *National Diet and Nutrition Survey: Young People Aged 4 to 18 Years*. London: The Stationery Office.

HEA (Health Education Authority) (1998) *Young and Active? Policy Framework for Young People and Health-Enhancing Physical Activity*. London: HEA.

Janz, K. F., Dawson, J. D. & Mahoney, L. T. (2000) Tracking physical fitness and physical activity from childhood to adolescence: The Muscatine Study, *Medicine and Science in Sports and Exercise*, **32**, 1250–7.

Joint Health Surveys Unit (1998) *Health Survey for England: The Health of Young People 1995–1997*. London: HMSO.

Malina, R. M. (1996) Tracking of physical activity and physical fitness across the lifespan, *Research Quarterly for Exercise and Sport*, **67**(supplement 3), 48–57.

Marshall, S. J., Biddle, S. J. H., Sallis, J. F., McKenzie, T. L. & Conway, T. L. (2002) Clustering of sedentary behaviours and physical activity among youth: a cross-national study, *Pediatric Exercise Science*, **14**, 401–17.

McAuley, E. & Mihalko, S. (1998) Measuring exercise related self-efficacy. In Duda, J. (ed), *Advances in Sport and Exercise Psychology Measurement*. Morgantown, WV: Fitness Information Technology, 371–90.

McElroy, M. (2002) *Resistance to Exercise: A Social Analysis of Inactivity*. Champaign, IL: Human Kinetics.

McLeroy, K., Bibeau, D., Steckler, A. & Glanz, K. (1988) An ecological perspective on health promotion programs, *Health Education Quarterly*, **15**(**4**), 351–77.

Morrow, J., Jackson, A. & Payne, V. (1999) Physical activity promotion and school physical education, *President's Council on Physical Fitness and Sports Research Digest*, **3**(**1**), 1–7.

Mulvihill, C., Rivers, K. & Aggleton, P. (2000) *Physical activity 'At Our Time'*. London: Health Education Authority.

Owen, N., Leslie, E., Salmon, J. & Fotheringham, M. J. (2000) Environmental determinants of physical activity and sedentary behaviour, *Exercise and Sport Science Reviews*, **28**(**4**), 165–70.

Pate, R. R., Trost, S. G., Dowda, M., Ott, A. E., Ward, D. S., Saunders, R. & Felton, G. (1999) Tracking of physical activity, physical inactivity, and health-related physical fitness in rural youth, *Pediatric Exercise Science*, **11**, 364–76.

Prochaska, J., Rodgers, M. & Sallis, J. (2002) Association of parent and peer support with adolescent physical activity, *Research Quarterly for Exercise and Sport*, **73**, 206–10.

Raitakari, O. T., Porkka, K. V. K., Taimela, S., Telama, R., Rasanen, L. & Viikari, J. S. A. (1994) Effects of persistent physical activity and inactivity on coronary risk factors in children and young adults: The Cardiovascular Risk in Young Finns Study, *American Journal of Epidemiology*, **140**, 195–205.

Resnicow, K., Robinson, T. & Frank, E. (1996) Advances and future directions for school-based health promotion research: commentary on the CATCH intervention trial, *Preventive Medicine* , **25**, 378–83.

Robinson, T. N. (1999) Reducing children's television viewing to prevent obesity, *Journal of the American Medical Association*, **282**(**16**), 1561–67.

Saelens, B., Sallis, J. & Frank, L. (2003) Environmental correlates of walking and cycling: findings from the transportation, urban design, and planning literatures, *Annals of Behavioral Medicine*, **25**, 80–91.

Sallis, J. (2000) Age-related decline in physical activity: a synthesis of human and animal studies, *Medicine and Science in Sports and Exercise*, **32**, 1597–1600.

Sallis, J., Bauman, A. & Pratt, M. (1998) Environmental and policy interventions to promote physical activity, *American Journal of Preventive Medicine*, **15**, 379–97.

Sallis, J., Kraft, K. & Linton, L. (2002) How the environment shapes physical activity: a transdisciplinary research agenda, *American Journal of Preventive Medicine*, **22(3)**, 208.

Sallis, J. & Owen, N. (1997) Ecological Models. In Glanz, K., Lewis, F. & Rimer, B. (eds), *Health Behavior and Health Education: Theory, Research and Practice*, 2nd edn. San Francisco, CA: Jossey-Bass, 403–24.

Sallis, J. & Owen, N. (1999) *Physical Activity and Behavioral Medicine*. Thousand Oaks, CA: Sage.

Sallis, J. & Owen, N. (2002) Ecological models of health behavior. In Glanz, K., Rimer, B. & Lewis, F. (eds), *Health Behavior and Health Education: Theory, Research and Practice*, 3rd edn. San Francisco, CA: Jossey Bass, 462–84.

Sallis, J., Prochaska, J. & Taylor, W. (2000) A review of correlates of physical activity of children and adolescents, *Medicine and Science in Sports and Exercise*, **32**, 963–75.

Schmitz, K. H., Lytle, L. A., Phillips, G. A., Murray, D. M., Birnbaum, A. S. & Kubik, M. Y. (2002) Psychosocial correlates of physical activity and sedentary leisure habits in young adolescents: The Teens Eating for Energy at School Study, *Preventive Medicine*, **34(2)**.

Smedley, B. & Syme, S. (eds) (2000) *Promoting Health: Intervention Strategies from Social and Behavioral Sciences*. Washington, D.C.: National Academy Press.

Spence, J. & Lee, R. (2003) Toward a comprehensive model of physical activity, *Psychology of Sport and Exercise*, **4**, 7–24.

Stokols, D. (1992) Establishing and maintaining healthy environments: towards a social ecology of health promotion, *American Psychologist*, **47**, 6–22.

Stone, E., McKenzie, T., Welk, G. & Booth, M. (1998) Effects of physical activity interventions in youth: review and synthesis, *American Journal of Preventive Medicine*, **15**, 298–315.

Vara, L. S. & Epstein, L. H. (1993) Laboratory assessment of choice between exercise or sedentary behaviors, *Research Quarterly for Exercise and Sport*, **64**, 356–60.

Vilhjalmsson, R. & Kristjansdottir, G. (2003) Gender differences in physical activity in older children and adolescents: the central role of organized sport, *Social Science and Medicine*, **56**, 363–74.

Wechsler, H., Devereaux, R., Davis, M. & Collins, J. (2000) Using the school environment to promote physical activity and healthy eating, *Preventive Medicine*, **31**(supplement), S121–37.

Wold, B. & Hendry, L. (1998) Social and environmental factors associated with physical activity in young people. In Biddle, S., Sallis, J. & Cavill, N. (eds), *Young and Active? Young People and Health-Enhancing Physical Activity – Evidence and Implications*. London: Health Education Authority, 119–32.

WHO (World Health Organisation) (2000) Health and Health Behaviour among Young People. WHO Policy Series: *Health Policy for Children and Adolescents*, Issue 1. Copenhagen: WHO.

5

Exercise Recommendations for Young People

Lorraine Cale and Jo Harris

Attempts to promote physical activity in young people should be based on well-established physical activity guidelines (Corbin & Pangrazi, 1999). However, whilst there is strong international consensus on the amount and type of physical activity that is beneficial to adult health, and much progress has been made in the promotion of physical activity among adults, the same cannot be said for young people for whom the evidence base is weaker (HEA, 1998a). For a number of years, the research foundation for the prescribed quantity and quality of exercise for young people was based on studies conducted on adults, and adult recommendations tended to be applied to children with no clear rationale (Cale & Harris, 1993; 1996; 2001; Pate, Trost & Williams, 1998). In the last ten years, however, a good deal of effort has been put into the development of physical activity guidelines for children and adolescents (Twisk, 2001) and a number of exercise recommendations have been proposed specifically for young people, based on the most up-to-date scientific evidence and expertise available. In the first instance, these recommendations emanated from the US, but, as Laventure (1998) noted, they received little exposure in the UK. This was of some concern as, in order to promote physical activity effectively and offer young people appropriate and accurate advice about how much physical activity is beneficial, all concerned need to be informed about the latest developments in exercise prescription research.

More recently, physical activity guidelines have been developed within the UK (HEA, 1998a; Scottish Executive, 2003). The first comprehensive recommendations to be made were developed in England by the HEA (now the Health Development Agency) in 1998, and, in 2003, physical activity guidelines for young people were proposed in Scotland as part of their National Physical Activity Strategy, *Let's Make Scotland More Active* (Scottish Executive, 2003).

This chapter provides an overview of the major developments in exercise recommendations for young people in recent years, and, in particular, focuses on the guidelines to emanate from the UK. The UK recommendations are discussed and their practical application considered. In addition, some general limitations and cautions concerning young people's physical activity guidelines are highlighted.

Discussion point   What message(s) do you feel young people should be given concerning how much and what type of physical activity to do? What factors might influence the message(s)?

Exercise recommendations for young people – North American developments

Exercise recommendations for young people were first formulated and published in the US in the late 1970s and early 1980s (Pate & Blair, 1978; Rowland, 1981; Haskell, Montoye & Orenstein, 1985; ACSM, 1986; Riopel et al., 1986). These early recommendations mirrored those for adults and implied that, on the whole, the same general guidelines could be applied to both groups. It was known, for example, that training effects in children would occur if the adult-fitness formula was applied. The earliest formal guidance for young people was provided by the ACSM in 1988. As a result of increasing concern about young people's physical fitness, the ACSM published an Opinion statement on physical fitness in children and youth, the aim being to provide direction on the structure and scope of physical fitness programmes for young people (ACSM, 1988). This statement is summarized in Table 5.1.

In 1991, the ACSM expanded its recommendations to include practical advice for those involved in designing training programmes for children. The guidelines were to increase the quantity of exercise gradually, to ensure adequate muscular strength and flexibility, proper body mechanics and the use of proper footwear and appropriate running surfaces, and also to take appropriate precautions in high temperature environments (ACSM, 1991).

Table 5.1 Exercise recommendations for young people

Author/Year	Opinion statement on physical fitness in children and youth (ACSM, 1988)	The Children's Lifetime Physical Activity Model (Cobin, Pangrazi & Welk, 1994)		Physical Activity Guidelines for Adolescents (Sallis & Patrick, 1994)	
Target group	Children and Youth	Children		Adolescents (11–21 years)	
		Minimum	Optimal	Guideline 1	Guideline 2
Frequency	Every day	Daily, 3 or more sessions a day	Daily, 3 or more sessions a day	Daily or nearly every day	3 or more sessions a week
Intensity	Vigorous	Moderate (to expend at least 3 kcal/kg/day)	Moderate to vigorous (to expend at least 6–8 kcal/kg/day)	Intensity not as important as fact that energy is expended	Moderate to vigorous
Time	20–30 minutes	30 minutes or more	60 minutes or more	Time not as important as fact that energy is expended	20 minutes or longer
Type		Childhood games and lifestyle activities (e.g. walking to school)	Childhood games, lifestyle activities and a variety of enjoyable activities which use large muscle groups and include some weight bearing	Variety of activities which are enjoyable, involve a range of muscle groups and include some weight bearing activities	Range of activities using large muscle groups

Following these initial recommendations, efforts were made to move away from 'adult-like' guidelines for fitness, to prescriptions which would promote short-term goals and enhance future health and wellbeing. Thus, in acknowledgement of the limitations of using adult guidelines with children, the Children's Lifetime Physical Activity Model (Corbin, Pangrazi & Welk, 1994) was proposed, the details of which are presented in Table 5.1. Within this model, both minimal and optimal levels of physical activity were recommended. Evidence suggests that, among adults, three to four kcal/kg/day is a minimum standard for producing health benefits, and Corbin, Pangrazi & Welk (1994) decided that a similar standard for children seemed appropriate. They considered it to be a standard that inactive children should be able to achieve with a modest commitment to childhood games and lifestyle activities. The optimal level proposed was based on the notion that it was not unreasonable to establish such a goal for children since they have the time and energy for activity above minimum standards, provided that they see a reason to be active (Corbin, Pangrazi & Welk, 1994).

Also in 1994, the International Consensus Conference on Physical Activity Guidelines for Adolescents was convened to develop physical activity guidelines for adolescents (Sallis & Patrick, 1994). The guidelines presented were based on a systematic review of the scientific paediatric literature and represented the most informed guidelines that could be developed at that time (Sallis & Patrick, 1994) (see Table 5.1). It was acknowledged that the optimal amount of physical activity for health was not known but it was stressed that the guidelines were developed to provide an amount of physical activity that was adequate for health maintenance for the general population of adolescents (Sallis & Patrick, 1994). In contrast to previous exercise guidelines, the intensity or duration of the activity was not emphasised in guideline one, the rationale being that these are probably less important than the fact that energy is expended and a habit of daily activity established. Rather, this guideline focused on encouraging adolescents to incorporate physical activity into their lifestyles (e.g. by using stairs, walking or riding a bike). The basis for the guideline was that daily weight-bearing activities are critical for enhancing bone development that affects skeletal health throughout life, and substantial daily energy expenditure is expected to reduce risk of obesity and may also have other positive health effects (Sallis & Patrick, 1994). In guideline two, moderate to vigorous activities were described as those that required at least as much effort as brisk or fast walking. The rationale provided for this guideline was that regular participation in continuous moderate to vigorous activity during adolescence enhances psychological health, increases HDL cholesterol and increases cardiorespiratory fitness (Sallis & Patrick, 1994).

The Children's Lifetime Physical Activity Model (Corbin, Pangrazi & Welk, 1994) provided the basis for the development of further and more recent recommendations in the US. Following an extensive review over a three-year period, COPEC (the Council on Physical Education for Children), a council within NASPE (the National Association for Sports and Physical Education), developed a set of physical activity guidelines for preadolescent school-aged children, to complement the guidelines for adolescents (Sallis & Patrick, 1994). The guidelines represent a series of different recommendations and are supported with guidance on how they can be adapted to meet the needs of children aged five to nine and ten to 12 years (COPEC, 1998). It was hoped that they would be viewed as a good beginning point for separating expectations for children from those of adults or adolescents (Corbin & Pangrazi, 1999). The guidelines are summarized in Table 5.2.

Again, each guideline was supported with a rationale. For example, for guidelines one and two it was suggested that children require more activity than adults because they are inherently active, need activity for normal growth and development, and need time in activity to develop lifetime physical activity skills. Furthermore, they need to focus on developing all parts of health-related physical fitness. Intermittent exercise was proposed in guideline three because children have a short attention span, are concrete rather than abstract thinkers, and are therefore not captivated by continuous vigorous activity. Also, they are intermittently active by nature and evidence suggests that intermittent exercise is necessary for normal growth (Pate, Corbin & Pangrazi, 1998).

Exercise recommendations for young people in the UK

Exercise recommendations for young people in England

In 1997, and in response to concerns that the evidence base relating to young people and physical activity was relatively weak, the HEA began to initiate a process of expert consultation and a review of the evidence surrounding the promotion of health-enhancing physical activity for young people (Biddle, Sallis & Cavill, 1998). The intention was to produce a policy framework from a public health perspective, that would maximize the opportunity for young people in England to participate in and benefit

Table 5.2   Physical activity guidelines for children: a summary

Guideline 1 Primary school-aged children should accumulate at least *30 to 60 minutes* of age- and developmentally-appropriate physical activity from a variety of physical activities on all or most days of the week.
Guideline 2 An accumulation of *more than 60 minutes and up to several hours per day* of age and developmentally appropriate activity is encouraged for primary school-aged children.
Guideline 3 Some of the child's physical activity each day should be in periods lasting 10 to 15 minutes or more and include moderate-to-vigorous physical activity. This activity will typically be intermittent in nature involving alternating moderate to vigorous activity with *brief periods* of rest and recovery.
Guideline 4 *Extended periods of inactivity are inappropriate* for children.
Guideline 5 A variety of physical activities are recommended for primary school children.

from a lifetime of regular, health-enhancing physical activity. Experts in the field were commissioned to prepare a series of review papers on key aspects relating to physical activity and young people, and drafts of these papers were presented to over fifty academics and experts at a two-day symposium held in June 1997. These papers, which have since been published (Biddle, Sallis & Cavill, 1998), included a critique of existing guidelines for physical activity in young people (Pate, Trost & Williams, 1998). Based on the research and critique presented at this meeting, recommendations were made and a draft policy was prepared and issued for consultation. Following the consultation process, the final policy framework, *Young and Active?* (HEA, 1998a), was published in June 1998. It provides an up-to-date review of the evidence available and guidelines on the recommended level and type of physical activity for young people aged 5–18 years. By so doing, it aims to inform the work of all those involved in promoting health-enhancing physical activity with young people. Primary and secondary recommendations are proposed within the policy framework and these, as well as their rationales, are presented in Table 5.3.

Table 5.3   Recommendations for young people and physical activity in England

Recommendations	Rationale	Examples/Suggested activities
Primary		
All young people should participate in physical activity (PA) of at least moderate intensity for *one hour per day* Young people who currently do little activity should participate in PA of at least moderate intensity for *at least half an hour per day*	• Most young people are currently doing 30 minutes of moderate PA per day on most days • Childhood overweight and obesity is increasing • Many young people possess at least one modifiable risk factor • Many young people have symptoms of psychological distress	• Brisk walking, cycling, swimming, most sports, dance – carried out as part of transportation, physical education, games, sport, recreation, work or structured exercise or for younger children as part of active play – performed in a continuous fashion or accumulated throughout the day
Secondary		
At least twice a week, some of these activities should help to enhance and maintain muscular strength and flexibility and bone health	• Participation in strength and weight-bearing activities is positively associated with bone mineral density and can be related to reduced risk of osteoporosis	• Strength-enhancing activities: play (climbing, skipping, jumping), structured exercise (body conditioning, resistance exercises)

Table 5.3   (Continued)

Recommendations	Rationale	Examples/Suggested activities
	• Muscular strength is required to perform activities of daily life (e.g. lifting, carrying, bending, twisting) • Trunk strength and muscular flexibility may be associated with reduced risk of back pain in later life	• Weight-bearing activities: gymnastics, dance, aerobics, skipping, and sports such as basketball

Source: HEA, 1998a.

Exercise recommendations for young people in Scotland

In June 2001 Scottish ministers set up a National Physical Activity Task Force following a commitment in the Government's White Paper 'Towards a Healthier Scotland'. The aim of the task force was to develop a National Physical Activity Strategy. Following consultation, the strategy, *Let's Make Scotland More Active*, was published in February 2003, with the goal of increasing and maintaining the proportion of physically active people in Scotland (Scottish Executive, 2003). The target for young people is that 80 per cent of all children aged 16 and under meet the minimum recommended levels of physical activity by 2022. The strategy acknowledges that for young people the well-accepted health message is that 'Children should accumulate (build up) at least one hour of moderate activity on most days of the week' (Scottish Executive, 2003).

Moderate activity is defined as activity that uses about five to seven calories a minute – the equivalent of brisk walking. Further, the strategy cites a recent physical activity conference in which it was decided that, in order of priority, the emphasis should be as follows:

be active most days;
moderate activities are good for you;
be active for . . . one hour if you are a child or young person. (Scottish Executive, 2003)

The implied rationale for the guideline is that the WHO (World Health Organisation) supports it and one hour a day is the minimum needed to provide direct health benefits, learn and practise a wide range of activities, and live actively as a daily habit (Scottish Executive, 2003).

Practical application of the UK recommendations

Recently, reviews of physical activity guidelines for young people have been published (Cale & Harris, 2001; Twisk, 2001) which have raised issues, highlighted cautions and proposed recommendations concerning the implementation and/or future direction of guidelines. Twisk's (2001) paper, which represents a critical review of physical activity guidelines for young people, highlights confusion in the field and provides a critical interpretation of the rationale behind proposed guidelines. Cale & Harris's (2001) review, meanwhile, critiques and considers the practical application of the HEA recommendations. These reviews are relevant when considering the practical application of both the HEA's (HEA, 1998a) and Scotland's Physical Activity Task Force guidelines (Scottish Executive, 2003).

Strengths

Certainly, the publication of age and culturally appropriate recommendations by the HEA and the Scottish Executive are most welcome and signal significant progress in the field of exercise prescription for young people. Furthermore, although the sets of guidelines have their differences, the common focus and message of one hour of moderate physical activity provides common ground for all those working to increase young people's levels of physical activity within the UK.

In considering the utility of any recommendations, of importance is that they are realistic and attainable by the population for which they are intended (Cale & Harris, 2001). On this issue, in developing their recommendations, the HEA (1998a) explains how they were intended to take into account the current physical activity patterns and lifestyles of young people, so that they represented attainable goals. Further, by shifting the emphasis from vigorous towards moderate physical activity, the recommendations are not only more attainable but are in keeping with adult guidelines, which likewise promote participation in regular, moderate physical activity (HEA, 1994; Scottish Executive, 2003). Indeed, as Cale & Harris (2001) pointed out in their review, it is hoped that the message that physical activity does not have to be strenuous for benefits to be gained will make the prospect of participating more appealing to young people.

An additional attractive feature of the HEA guidelines, and in keeping with the Children's Lifetime Physical Activity Model and the Guidelines for Adolescents, is that they allow for differentiation within the recommendation (Cale & Harris, 2001). For example, although the aim is for all young people to be active for one hour per day, those who currently do little are advised to aim for half an hour per day. Within the Scottish recommendations, a degree of differentiation and flexibility is implied by their suggestion that there is an order of priority of emphasis within the recommendation (Scottish Executive, 2003) (see earlier).

It is also noteworthy that the HEA and the Scottish Executive guidelines have adopted the term 'physical activity' rather than 'exercise' within their recommendations. Evidence suggests that many people's perceptions of exercise, including the young, are that it involves hard work, effort, strenuous activities, gyms and organized sports, and is often considered to be unattractive, irrelevant or even intimidating (HEA, 1994; 1998b). Indeed, the HEA's definition of exercise as 'planned, structured and repetitive bodily movement done to improve or maintain one or more components of physical fitness' (HEA, 1998a, p. 2) is unlikely to sound appealing to young people. Physical activity, on the other hand, which is described as 'a broad term to describe movement of the body that uses energy' involving 'exercise, sport, play, dance and active living such as walking, housework and gardening' (HEA, 1998a, p. 8) is all-encompassing and likely to be more attractive and relevant.

Similarly, the shift to accumulating physical activity over the course of the day is considered to be more attainable and relevant, particularly for younger children. As Chapter 2 revealed, research has consistently shown that continuous, sustained exercise is not a feature of children's exercise behaviour and that young people's physical activity tends to be sporadic and consist of relatively short bouts of intense activity (Bailey et al., 1995; Armstrong & Van Mechelen 1998). As a consequence, elements of previous guidelines which have advocated sustained physical activity, and particularly those prescribing durations of 20 minutes or more (ACSM, 1988; Sallis & Patrick, 1994), are now considered inappropriate for many young people.

A further point to note concerning the utility of the UK recommendations is the degree of flexibility that is afforded within them. The aim is for young people to be active daily but acknowledgement is made by the HEA that physical activity can vary from day to day in type, setting, intensity, duration and amount, and that the methods of meeting the recommendations may also vary according to stage of maturation. For example, it is considered that many young children are likely to achieve the primary recommendation during play, whereas some teenagers are more likely to achieve it by participating in more structured continuous bouts of moderate to vigorous physical activity. Scotland's Physical Activity Strategy similarly identifies the wide range of activities that young people can access, including play, dance, exercise, outdoor activities, active travel, as well as the different settings in which they can be active (e.g. the home, school, community) (Scottish Executive, 2003).

The National Physical Activity Strategy for Scotland acknowledges evidence that shows that the physical activity message is a complicated one, comprising time, intensity and frequency. It suggests, therefore, that is it necessary to communicate it to the public and policy-makers as simply as possible (Scottish Executive, 2003). By comparison with previous guidelines, however, and with reference to the HEA recommendations, Cale & Harris (2001) argue to the contrary that the UK recommendations are presented in relatively 'user' and 'child friendly' language. Concerns have been expressed in the past over the limited utility of overly technical prescriptions (Simons-Morton et al., 1988) and precise, accurate and scientific exercise prescriptions are of little use if few want to, or indeed are able to, follow them. Historically, for example, some guidelines have advocated that physical activity intensity should be between a specific percentage of maximum heart rate (e.g. 60–90 per cent for fitness; 55–90 per cent for health) (ACSM, 1990; 1991), or should elicit a heart rate above a particular threshold (e.g. >140 beats per minute) (Simons-Morton et al., 1988). Cale & Harris (1996; 2001) suggest that concepts relating to intensity may be difficult for young people to grasp, and it would therefore seem wise to adopt a simpler, clearer message relating to the effort involved. Both UK guidelines have adopted a clear message, recommending activities of at least moderate intensity, defined as activity usually equivalent to brisk walking, which might be expected to leave the participant feeling warm and slightly out of breath (HEA, 1998a), or as activity which uses about five to seven calories a minute – the equivalent of brisk walking (Scottish Executive, 2003).

A particularly positive development within the HEA recommendation is considered to be the introduction of activities to promote a range of components of physical fitness, namely muscular strength and endurance and flexibility, as well as aerobic fitness (Cale & Harris, 2001). By including strength and flexibility within a secondary recommendation, this is the first time for children that these components have been formally included within a specific guideline. Guideline five of the Physical Activity Guidelines for Children acknowledges participation in activities that develop strength, muscular endurance and flexibility, but they are not recognized as a guideline in their own right. Muscular strength and flexibility exercises have the potential to provide numerous benefits to young people, including enhanced performance, improved posture, reduced risk of injury and protection against future back pain and osteoporosis (Plowman, 1992; Grimston, Willows & Hanley, 1993). Muscular strength and endurance and flexibility are often neglected components of physical fitness and a specific recommendation to promote these aspects represents good practice. In addition, and as a consequence, it may mean that young people are offered and encouraged to engage in a broad, balanced and varied exercise programme that may in turn help to sustain their motivation and interest (Cale & Harris, 2001).

A final significant feature of the guidelines is that both are supported by further recommendations, goals and/or priorities signalling how they might be achieved. The HEA policy framework presents a series of recommendations which focus on the role of key organizations in promoting physical activity for young people (HEA, 1998a). The framework identifies the education sector (including schools, further and higher education colleges, youth services, local education authorities, advisory and support services, and professional bodies), the health services (including health promotion, primary health care and directors of public health), local authorities, organizations concerned with sport and recreation and/or young people, mass media and government departments as having a vital role to play in promoting health-enhancing physical activity for young people. Common themes within the recommendations for all organizations are the importance of adopting a holistic approach to physical activity promotion and on developing and working in partnerships. Furthermore, the HEA recognize the need to focus specifically on the inactive, and identify girls aged 12–18 years, young people of low socio-economic status and older adolescents as priority groups for physical activity interventions.

Given that the guidelines for Scotland are contained within a National Physical Activity Strategy, these are naturally supported by specific goals, strategic objectives and priorities. In order to bring about changes in physical activity levels, the strategy identifies strategic priorities for life-stage groups and settings. For children and young people, it states that special efforts are needed to ensure that action responds to those in greatest need and in particular to teenage girls.

Furthermore, and as with *Young and Active?*, the strategy acknowledges that there are many different national agencies that could help put the objectives and priorities into practice and advocates the need for an identifiable and accountable cross-cutting (joined-up) structure (Scottish Executive, 2003). It identifies a range of local services including local government (transport and planning; education; leisure, recreation and culture; social services, etc.), the NHS, health boards, voluntary organizations, local enterprise companies and businesses and other organizations (such as universities and colleges, housing associations, media, community safety) and the possible contributions they could make in helping to achieve physical activity objectives.

Limitations

The UK recommendations undoubtedly represent a significant and welcomed development. However, they, as with any young people guidelines, have their limitations and need to be interpreted and employed with some degree of caution. Twisk (2001) reminds us that the scientific evidence on which such guidelines are based is rather weak and suggests that the field is confused and controversial, and the guidelines highly speculative. For guidelines to be developed, he explains, there has to be a relationship between physical activity and health and the relationship has to have a certain shape on which to base the guidelines (e.g. linear, hyperbolic, parabolic, s-shaped). However, there is only marginal evidence that physical activity is beneficial for health during childhood and adolescence, and hardly any evidence that these health benefits have some sort of threshold value. Twisk (2001) recommends, therefore, that guidelines should perhaps focus on aspects other than possible health benefits. Indeed, Blair et al. (1989) have suggested that activity guidelines should focus primarily on the establishment of activity habits, which, according to Rowland (1996), avoids the thorny question of how much activity is necessary and the temptation to adopt definitive guidelines based on weak and inconsistent evidence. Indeed, in recognition of this, Health Canada and the Canadian Society for Exercise Physiology recently made the decision not to propose an empirical recommendation. Instead, they initiated the development of physical activity 'guides' and supporting resources for children and youth. The guides were launched in April 2002 and promote the messages that children and youth should increase their physical activity by a total of at least 30 minutes per day, and reduce 'non-active' time spent on TV, video, and computer games by at least 30 minutes per day (www.hc-sc.gc.ca/hppb/paguide).

In previous reviews, Cale & Harris (1993; 1996; 2001) highlighted a number of issues concerning the practical application of guidelines and cautioned that recommendations should:

- be guidelines, not strict rules, rigid prescriptions or unyielding standards;
- represent principles, 'not theorems or laws';
- be used with common sense and sensitivity;
- be viewed not as a starting point but as a goal towards which to progress;
- take into account young people's health and activity histories, physical fitness levels, functional capacities, personal circumstances, goals and preferences/dislikes.

In addition, they proposed the following key messages:

- All physical activity, performed safely, provides health benefits.
- Even very low-level physical activity (e.g. leisurely walking) is beneficial.
- Imposing standards on young people or forcing them to participate in a regime of physical activity should be avoided.
- Dictating the same starting point and rate of progression for all should be avoided.

In summary, Cale & Harris (2001) advocate that an individualized, personalized and differentiated approach should be adopted when giving physical activity guidance to young people. Young people should be respected and treated as individuals and helped to set individual, attainable, short-term goals and encouraged to engage in the types and amounts of physical activity which are appropriate for and appealing to them. No hierarchy of activities should exist in the promotion of physical activity and young people should learn to value all forms and types of physical activity.

On this note, the HEA recognize within their policy framework that 'young people are not a homogenous group' (HEA, 1998a, p. 6) and suggest that interventions should be differentiated on the grounds of gender, age/life-stage and socio-economic status, and that programmes should be designed to meet the specific needs of young people. Similarly, Scotland's National Physical Activity Strategy recognizes that community-planning partnerships need to identify and take account of local needs and priorities.

Concerning the recommended frequency and time of activity within the recommendations, it cannot be assumed that young people will be able to make time, will wish to, or will find suitable opportunities to exercise for one hour daily (Cale & Harris, 2001). This point was also acknowledged with reference to the Children's Lifetime Physical Activity Model and the Guidelines for Adolescents in which daily activity is also a key feature (Cale & Harris, 1996). The view of Corbin, Pangrazi & Welk (1994) that children have the time and energy for activity is arguable, especially for older children with school, home and possibly part-time work commitments. Time is a frequently cited barrier to exercise for many young people (Sallis, 1994; Mason, 1995; Mulvihill, Rivers & Aggleton, 2000). The intention within both sets of guidelines is that such activity may be performed continuously or accumulated throughout the day, but this is not altogether clear within the HEA recommendations. The guidelines for Scotland are more explicit and include (and qualify) the term 'accumulate' ('build up') within their recommendation.

Clearly, in encouraging young people to work towards the one hour recommendation, they will need to be helped to recognize the factors which constrain their physical activity participation (such as a lack of time, money, facilities, transport), and to overcome them. In addition, they will need to appreciate the broad and full range of physical activity opportunities available to them, and time-effective ways and means of incorporating such activities into their daily lives (e.g. walking or cycling to school, to the shops or to meet friends). Indeed, this should be addressed as part of the physical education and personal, social and health education curriculum in schools (see Chapter 7).

Still on the issue of time, Cale & Harris (2001) argue that engaging in less activity than that which is recommended does not mean that it will not be beneficial. Twisk (2001) also lends support to this notion. As already noted, the scientific basis for the guidelines is weak, and neither the minimal nor the optimal amount of physical activity for young people can be precisely defined at this time (HEA, 1998a; Twisk, 2001). Twisk (2001, p. 625) states:

> based on the present scientific evidence, the proposed guidelines are as valid as stating every increase in physical activity can have some beneficial health effects for children and adolescents. The advantage of such a simple guideline is that this goal is much easier to achieve than the 30 or 60 minutes of moderate intensity physical activity each day … [and] when reached, probably leads to the same health benefits as that achieved by the guideline goals proposed by the expert committees.

However, the HEA defend their recommendation, explaining that, until further research leads to refinements, expert opinion strongly supports the one hour recommendation (HEA, 1998a). Scotland's Physical Activity Strategy advocates this amount on account that this health message is well accepted and supported by the WHO (Scottish Executive, 2003).

Furthermore, it is argued that the rationale provided for 60 (as opposed to 30) minutes of moderate activity on most days (see Table 5.3) is flawed (Twisk, 2001). The argument given against a guideline for 30 minutes of moderate activity on most days of the week was that, although most young people are currently meeting this criterion, the incidence of overweight children and childhood obesity is increasing and many young people have been shown to possess at least one modifiable coronary heart disease risk factor (HEA, 1998a). Twisk (2001), however, notes that this argument ignores the fact that the aetiology of every chronic disease is highly multidimensional and not fully understood (in other words, the increased incidence of overweight children and childhood obesity and the existence of at least one modifiable cardiovascular disease risk factor is not *per se* caused by a decrease in physical activity), and the fact that there is only marginal evidence that physical activity is related to cardiovascular disease risk factors in children and adolescents (i.e. it is caused by factors other than a decrease in physical activity).

A further issue relates to how the recommendations are likely to be promoted, interpreted and accepted by young people as well as significant others (e.g. parents, teachers, health professionals). Evidence from Scotland's recent Health Education Population Survey (HEBS, 1998) revealed that only 34 per cent of the population were aware of the one hour, moderate physical activity message and a recent study which investigated the reported perceptions of, motivations for, and barriers to physical activity among young people revealed limited awareness of physical activity guidelines (Mulvihill, Rivers, & Aggleton, 2000). Meanwhile, a similar study involving 16-to-24-year-old young women (HEA, 1998b) revealed generally good awareness that exercise guidance existed, but uncertainty and scepticism about the messages. A number of questions were raised by subjects in the study about the precision, uniformity and validity of exercise guidelines. One young woman asked, 'does it need to be so precise – what if you do shorter periods more often?', and another commented that there were 'too many conflicting messages' (HEA, 1998b). It is therefore important that the scope and utility of exercise recommendations be discussed with young people and that they be made aware that, as helpful as formal guidelines are, they should not be taken as absolute and unyielding standards.

Laventure (1998) has also noted how in the past physical activity guidelines have received little exposure and had minimal impact in the UK. The same could be said of the HEA guidelines. For example, the recommendations still do not feature within the curriculum in most schools. Scotland's Physical Activity Strategy recognizes this issue and highlights education programmes and the media as effective ways of raising awareness (Scottish Executive, 2003).

The HEA should be applauded for including a secondary recommendation for the enhancement of muscular strength and flexibility and bone health. That said, it is suggested that this recommendation should be interpreted carefully and implemented with caution (Cale & Harris, 2001). There are some specific safety considerations in carrying out strength and flexibility work with young people and there are risks associated with some forms of strength and flexibility training. According to Harris (2000), these are mainly associated with unsupervised lifting of heavy weights and with extreme stretch positions. The intention in the HEA's recommendations is not that young children should be encouraged to perform 'adult-type' formal strength and flexibility exercises, but that modifications and alternate versions of these may be appropriate for adolescents. If considering recommending or incorporating structured strength and flexibility work with young people, it is important to be aware of guidelines relating to the amount and type they should be doing. Based on a review of the relevant literature, a series of recommendations have been made (Harris, 2000) which are outlined in Table 5.4. Further guidance on resistance training and young people is also soon to be published by the British Association of Sport and Exercise Sciences. The 'best practice' document identifies the evidence base regarding the

Table 5.4 Recommendations for strength and flexibility exercises with young people

---

Recommendations

Weight- or load-bearing activities are recommended for children of all ages. These include activities in which the body has to support (1) all or part of its own weight (e.g. running, jumping, dancing, gymnastics); (2) the weight of additional objects (e.g. a throwing or striking implement such as a bat, ball, bean bag, quoit, hoop).

Young children (4–11 year olds) should be involved in a wide range of weight-bearing activities for both the upper body (e.g. climbing, throwing, catching, striking) and the lower body (e.g. running, jumping, hopping, skipping). **Nine to eleven years olds** can additionally be involved in developmentally-appropriate low level exercises involving their own body weight such as 'easy' curl ups (with legs bent and hands along floor) for the abdominal ('tummy') muscles and 'easy' push ups (against a wall or in a box position) for muscles in the arms and chest.

Education about **back care** is important for **all children**. Safe lifting, carrying and lowering involves:

> getting close to the object being lifted
> keeping a wide solid base with feet apart and firmly on the ground
> using the large leg muscles rather than the back muscles
> tightening the abdominal muscles
> keeping the back straight when lifting or lowering
> holding the object close to the body
> getting assistance if the object is very heavy.

Older children (11 years and upwards) should be involved in differentiated exercises involving their own body weight, particularly for muscles which assist good posture (i.e. the back and abdominal muscles). **It is recommended that young people learn how to perform body resistance exercises with good technique before progressing on to exercises involving external weights**.

Low resistance external weights (such as light dumb-bells, elastics and tubing) can be safely used by older children (11 year olds and upwards). **Medium to high resistance external weights** (as is possible with fixed equipment such as a multi-gym and with free weights such as dumb-bells and barbells) are only advisable with 14–18 year olds. Lifting **near-maximal weights** is only appropriate for young people aged 16–18 years who have reached the final stage of maturation.

Each **strength exercise** should be performed no more than 10 times before resting the muscles involved. Unfamiliar exercises should be performed 4 to 6 times, progressing over time to 10 repeats. **Controlled lifting and lowering** should be emphasised. There should be gradual progression from 1 to 3 sets. Each session should include exercises for a balanced range of major muscle groups. No more than 3 sessions a week of strength exercises is recommended and there should be at least one day's rest between sessions. Any increases in frequency, intensity or duration should be gradual (by only 5–10% at a time).

Stretching exercises are recommended for all age groups, especially older children (11 years and upwards). Stretching should only be performed following cardiovascular activity when the muscles are warm. Each **stretch** should be moved into slowly and held still. The holding time for stretches should vary from 6 to 20 seconds (depending on the weather conditions, how warm the muscles are, and the age and maturity of the children). Young children (4–11 year olds) can learn simple and frequently-used stretches (e.g. whole body stretches; calf stretches) while older children can learn stretches for specific muscle groups (e.g. triceps, hamstrings). **It is recommended that stretches are taught within warm-ups and cool-downs**. The knowledge, understanding and skills associated with stretching should be progressively taught over time.

With reference to both strength and stretching exercises, the emphasis with all age groups should be on **safety and quality**, not quantity, with particular attention paid to **progression** and **balance**. Young people should understand the purpose of exercises and be able to perform them with good technique and at a developmentally-appropriate level (i.e. one which matches their stage of physical and psychological maturity). They should know how to make exercises easier or harder.

The **learning environment** should be positive and non-threatening and the focus should be on **personal improvement**, not comparison with others. The delivery should aim to involve young people in their own learning and promote a **responsible attitude** towards safe, health-enhancing exercise behaviour.

Properly designed strength and flexibility training programmes for young people should be:
(i)   child-centred and individualized, including developmentally-appropriate exercises which match the physical and psychological maturity of the young person
(ii) progressive with only gradual increases in frequency, intensity or duration being made at any one time

Table 5.4   (Continued)

Recommendations
(iii)   balanced (i.e. only one part of a total exercise programme; incorporating all the major muscle groups)
(iv)   competently taught and closely supervised by an appropriately qualified adult.

Source: Health-related Exercise in the National Curriculum Key Stages 1 to 4. Copyright © 2000 by Jo Harris. By permission of Human Kinetics, Champaign, IL, USA.

benefits (and risks) associated with the participation of young people in resistance training and includes consensus guidelines for the design and delivery of resistance exercise programmes for young people (Research into Exercise Activity and Children's Health (REACH) Group, in press).

In the authors' opinion, and as has been acknowledged elsewhere (Cale & Harris, 2001), more guidance should have been provided in support of the secondary recommendation to ensure that it is not misunderstood. In contrast, and in recognition of the importance of recommending developmentally appropriate activity for children, the most recent guidelines from the US (COPEC, 1998) provide details on how these can be adapted to meet the needs of children of different ages.

A further issue relates to the likely success of the key organizations identified in both the HEA policy framework and Scotland's National Physical Activity Strategy, in being able to fulfil their proposed role in promoting physical activity. For example, are all organizations aware of the contribution they can and should be making to achieving physical activity objectives? Secondly, do they have the knowledge and expertise, resources and time to successfully contribute and impact upon young people's physical activity levels? Thirdly, who is responsible and to whom are they accountable if they do not or cannot? Within the National Physical Activity Strategy, the Scottish Executive (2003) suggests that in the past there has been a lack of co-ordination and overall responsibility for physical activity and that what is needed is leadership, co-ordination and resources for a strategic approach.

Finally, in an attempt to address some of the key issues associated with exercise recommendations and young people, Cale & Harris (2001) provided a number of ideas for implementing or 'practically applying' the recommendations with young people (see Table 5.5). The content

Table 5.5   Ideas for implementing the recommendations

Issue	Implementation Idea
Key Concepts/Foci	• Ensure that the key concepts and main foci of planning, delivery and evaluation are health, participation and physical activity and are holistic and inclusive • Provide a structured programme which teaches all young people about the benefits and risks of physical activity and inactivity and provides them with opportunities to experience and learn through a broad and varied range of activities
Developmentally – appropriate Activity	• Consider and incorporate into planning and delivery the appropriateness of particular activities for differing maturity levels (e.g. full push-ups are inappropriate for young children (under 11 years) as well as for some older children) • Ensure that suitable alternatives are offered (e.g. climbing; gymnastic activities; 'easier' versions of exercises such as push-ups)
Flexibility/differentiation	• Provide choices within activities (e.g. of exercise type and level of intensity) • Do not put down young people who opt for less demanding versions of activities – be positive and encouraging

Table 5.5   (Continued)

Issue	Implementation Idea
Environment	• Focus feedback on personal progress and improvement, not on achievement in relation to others • Ensure that the physical activity environment is appealing (clean, warm, inviting) • Ensure the physical activity environment reflects an inclusive and holistic philosophy (e.g. posters portraying individuals of differing shapes, sizes, colours, abilities, disabilities, etc; equipment which caters for a range of abilities)
Encouragement/rewards	• Show interest in what physical activity young people do (in school and in their leisure time) • Offer and provide rewards (e.g. praise, treat) for increases in physical activity (e.g. joining in or helping out with a club or community event, including organizing, coaching and officiating) and also reductions in physical inactivity (e.g. watching less TV; spending less time playing on the computer)
Respect	• Listen and aim to respond to comments (positive and negative) made by young people about physical activity, sport, physical education and the activities offered to them (including in schools through the extended curriculum)

- Do not ignore persistent
  obstructive issues such as
  gender, unappealing
  activities, showering, PE
  kit (in school)
- Ask young people for
  their views, ideas and
  suggestions about current
  and future developments

Source: Cale & Harris (2001). Reprinted with permission.

was originally developed with the school curriculum in mind but all individuals involved in promoting physical activity in young people are encouraged to incorporate these ideas, as appropriate, into their work, and/or disseminate them to relevant others.

Case studies

Taking into account the current physical activity guidelines for young people and the discussion of their practical application, what physical activity guidance would you give to the following individuals?

1. Nick is an overweight 10-year-old who is very inactive. He claims that he dislikes PE and sport at school and spends most of his time watching TV, playing computer games or listening to music. He generally prefers his own company though has a couple of friends who live nearby.
2. Jo is a highly active teenager who regularly takes part in and enjoys most sports. She is a particularly keen swimmer and she trains most days and competes for her school and swimming club.
3. Tom, aged 17, does some, though limited, physical activity. He generally likes sport and exercise but school work and a part-time job mean that he has little leisure time.

Conclusions

The UK guidelines on the level and type of physical activity for young people published by the HEA (1998a) and the Scottish Executive

(2003) signal significant progress in the field and provide common ground and a common message for all those working to increase young people's physical activity levels. A number of positive features of the recommendations have been identified and it is considered that they are more realistic, flexible, appealing and attainable than previous recommendations. However, although the new guidelines provide a useful indicator as to the desirable volume of exercise for young people, the issues, limitations, cautions and key messages highlighted in reviews (Cale & Harris, 1993; 1996; 2001; Twisk, 2001) should be borne in mind, and further research and discussion is needed (Corbin & Pangrazi, 1999; Twisk, 2001). Twisk (2001) suggests that, in order to obtain guidelines for children and adolescents, experimental studies are needed in which groups of children and adolescents with different frequencies, modes and volumes of physical activity are compared with each other in relation to certain health outcomes. These experiments of course are difficult to perform. Until such a time, though, the value of physical activity guidelines for young people for public health purposes is beyond doubt and guidelines can be usefully employed in a number of ways to promote young people's current and future activity levels. However, much depends on their successful dissemination. Physical activity guidelines need to be widely promoted and made accessible and comprehensible to all involved in promoting physical activity in young people. To date in the UK, there is little evidence to suggest that this has happened. Future efforts clearly need to be directed towards bridging this policy–practice gap.

Discussion point What implications do the UK physical activity guidelines for young people have for:

1 you as an individual?
2 teachers of physical education/personal, social and health education?
3 health professionals?
4 exercise professionals?
5 sports coaches?
6 the media?
7 government departments (e.g. Department for Education and Skills; Department for Transport, Local Government and the Regions; Department of Culture, Media and Sport)?

References

ACSM (American College of Sports Medicine) (1986) *Guidelines for Graded Exercise Testing and Prescription*, 3rd edn. Philadelphia: Lea & Febiger.

ACSM (American College of Sports Medicine) (1988) Opinion statement on physical fitness in children and youth, *Medicine and Science in Sport and Exercise*, **20(4)**, 422–3.

ACSM (American College of Sports Medicine) (1990) Position stand on the recommended quantity and quality of exercise for developing and maintaining cardiorespiratory and muscular fitness in healthy adults, *Medicine and Science in Sport and Exercise*, **22**, 265–74.

ACSM (American College of Sports Medicine) (1991) *Guidelines for Exercise Testing and Prescription*, 4th edn. Philadelphia: Lea & Febiger.

Armstrong, N. & Van Mechelen, W. (1998) Are young people fit and active? In Biddle, S., Sallis, J. & Cavill, N. (eds), *Young and Active? Young People and Health-Enhancing Physical Activity – Evidence and Implications*. London: Health Education Authority, 69–97.

Bailey, R. C., Olson, J., Pepper, S. L., Porszaz, J., Barstow, T. L. & Cooper, D. M. (1995) The level and tempo of children's physical activities: an observation study, *Medicine and Science in Sports and Exercise*, **27**, 1033–41.

Biddle, S., Sallis, J. F. & Cavill, N. (eds) (1998) *Young and Active? Young People and Health-Enhancing Physical Activity – Evidence and Implications*. London: Health Education Authority.

Blair, S. N., Clark, D. G., Cureton, K. J. & Powell, K. E. (1989) Exercise and fitness in childhood: implications for a lifetime of health. In Gisolfi, C. V. & Lamb, D. R. (eds), *Perspectives in Exercise Science and Sports Medicine*. Indianapolis, IN: Benchmark Press, 401–30.

Cale, L. & Harris, J. (1993) Exercise recommendations for children and young people, *Physical Education Review*, **16(2)**, 89–98.

Cale, L. & Harris, J. (1996) Understanding and evaluating the value of exercise guidelines for children. In Lidor, R., Eldar, E. & Harari, I. (eds), *Proceedings of the 1995 AIESEP World Congress: Bridging the Gaps Between Disciplines, Curriculum and Instruction*. Netanya, Israel: Wingate, 161–6.

Cale, L. & Harris, J. (2001) Exercise recommendations for young people: an update, *Health Education*, **101(3)**, 126–38.

COPEC (Council on Physical Education for Children). (1998) *Physical Activity for Children: A Statement of Guidelines*. Reston, VA: NASPE Publications.

Corbin, C. & Pangrazi, R. P. (1999) Physical activity for children: in pursuit of appropriate guidelines, *European Journal of Physical Education*, **4**, 139–45.

Corbin, C. B., Pangrazi, R. P. & Welk, G. J. (1994) Toward an understanding of appropriate physical activity levels for youth, *Physical Activity and Fitness Research Digest*, **Series 1(8)**, 1–7.

Grimston, S. K., Willows, N. D. & Hanley, D. A. (1993) Mechanical loading regime and its relationship to bone mineral density in children, *Medicine and Science in Sports and Exercise*, **25(11)**, 1203–20.

Harris, J. (2000) *Health-Related Exercise in the National Curriculum. Key Stages 1 to 4.* Champaign, IL: Human Kinetics.

Haskell, W. L., Montoye, H. J. & Orenstein, D. (1985) Physical activity and exercise to achieve health-related physical fitness components, *Public Health Report*, **100**, 202–12.

HEA (Health Education Authority) (1994) *Moving On: International Perspectives on Promoting Physical Activity*. London: HEA.

HEA (Health Education Authority) (1998a). *Young and Active? Policy Framework for Young People and Health-Enhancing Physical Activity*. London: HEA.

HEA (Health Education Authority) (1998b) *Physical Activity 'What We Think.' Qualitative Research among Women aged 16 to 24*. London: HEA.

HEBS (Health Education Board for Scotland) (1998) *Health Education Population Study*. Edinburgh: HEBS.

Laventure, B. (1998) Young and active? The development of a policy framework for young people and physical activity, *The British Journal of Physical Education*, **29(1)**, 33–4.

Mason, V. (1995) *Young People and Sport in England, 1994: A National Survey*. London: Sports Council.

Mulvihill, C., Rivers, K. & Aggleton, P. (2000) *Physical Activity 'At Our Time': Qualitative Research Among Young People Aged 5 to 15 Years and Parents*. London: Health Education Authority.

Pate, R. R. & Blair, S. N. (1978) Exercise and the prevention of atherosclerosis: pediatric implications. In Strong, W. (ed.), *Pediatric Aspects of Atherosclerosis*. New York: Grune & Stratton, 251–86.

Pate, R., Corbin, C. & Pangrazi, R. (1998) Physical activity for young people, *President's Council on Physical Fitness and Sports Research Digest*, **3(3)**, 1–6.

Pate, R., Trost, S. & Williams, C. (1998) Critique of existing guidelines for physical activity in young people. In Biddle, S., Sallis, J. & Cavill, N. (eds), *Young and Active? Young People and Health-enhancing Physical Activity – Evidence and Implications*. London: Health Education Authority, 162–73.

Plowman, S. A. (1992) Physical activity, physical fitness, and low back pain, *Exercise and Sport Sciences Reviews*, **20**, 21–242.

Research into Exercise Activity and Children's Health (REACH) Group. Liverpool John Moores University (in press) *Guidelines for Resistance Exercise in Young People*. Leeds: British Association of Sport and Exercise Sciences.

Riopel, D. A., Boerth, R. C., Coates, T. J., Hennekens, C. H., Miller, W. W. et al. (1986) Coronary risk factor modification in children: exercise, *Circulation*, **74**, 1189A–1191A.

Rowland, T. W. (1981) Physical fitness in children: implications for the prevention of coronary artery disease. In Gluck, L. (ed.), *Current Problems in*

Pediatrics, **11(9)**, 1–54. Medical Publications, Chicago: Year Book Medical Publishers.

Rowland, T. W. (1996) Is there a scientific rationale supporting the value of exercise for the present and future cardiovascular health of children? The con argument, *Pediatric Exercise Science*, **8**, 303–9.

Sallis, J. (1994) Influences on physical activity of children, adolescents, and adults or determinants of active living. *Physical Activity and Fitness Research Digest*, **Series 1(7)**, 1–8.

Sallis, J. F. & Patrick, K. (1994) Physical activity guidelines for adolescents: consensus statement, *Pediatric Exercise Science*, **6**, 302–14.

Scottish Executive (2003) *Let's Make Scotland More Active. A Strategy for Physical Activity. Physical Activity Task Force.* Edinburgh: The Stationery Office.

Simons-Morton, B. G., Parcel, G. S., O'Hara, N. M., Blair, S. N. & Pate, R. R. (1988) Health-related physical fitness in childhood: status and recommendations, *Annual Review of Public Health*, **9**, 403–25.

Twisk, J. W. R. (2001) Physical activity guidelines for children and adolescents. A critical review, *Sports Medicine*, **31(8)**, 617–27.

6

Models and Approaches in Exercise Promotion

Jim McKenna and Chris Riddoch

Theoretical models are important in the promotion of exercise because they help to show how and where physical activity interventions can best be developed. Of course, they do not often directly address the delivery of interventions, but instead provide strong clues about the important elements of their delivery. However, their relatively low predictive power, and what some may feel is their low capacity to initiate change, underlines the incompleteness of contemporary models. Furthermore, and as becomes evident within this chapter, relatively little attention has been paid to their application to young people.

Beginning with what seem to be the dominant models of exercise or physical activity behaviour change, this chapter describes their key components and theoretical features, and then progresses to address a range of the contemporary theoretical and practical concerns. This involves a shift from psychological theories to social perspectives. By so doing, the aim is to highlight useful opportunities for innovative developments in both theory and practice.

Existing models of behaviour change work on the basis of understanding how change might be best achieved – Schneider Jamner's (2000) 'leverage points'. They often capitalize on diverse perspectives that each contribute to physical activity involvement, meaning that practitioners often take the best from the different approaches to develop their own practice. Not surprisingly, practitioners see substantial overlap, whereas theoreticians see the need for careful definitions and distinctive ways of operationalizing their constructs.

Psychological and psychosocially-derived approaches

A common clarion call for researchers commenting on intervention design is to urge more theoretically-derived interventions (e.g. Freudenberg et al., 1995). The theories that are most recommended in such calls are those that reflect psychology and social psychology. Focus falls on these theories in this chapter since they relate most to individual health and physical activity promoters (and indeed to physical educators), whose practice is limited to interactions with individuals or small groups. Their professional lives may not be characterized by access to larger teams of professionals, nor by feeling central to community programmes. Beginning with the Transtheoretical Model (TTM) and the generic themes it proposes, the key features of the Social Cognitive Theory (SCT) and the Theory of Reasoned Action/Theory of Planned Behaviour (TPB/TRA) are then identified and critiqued.

The Transtheoretical Model

The Transtheoretical Model (TTM) claims to be a generic theory that subsumes many others, although it may also be seen as a decision-making theory (Biddle & Nigg, 2000). Derived from self-help for cessation behaviours such as smoking or drinking (Prochaska & DiClemente, 1982), the model has a strong record of positive outcome effects. Self-help is a preferred approach for behaviour change in many individuals (Garfield 1994; O' Connell, 1998), including for physical activity among young people (Klar, Nadler & Malloy, 1992). Based on 81 effect sizes from 40 separate general health studies, a meta-analytic review of self-administered treatment found positive programme effects over controls (Scogin et al., 1990) in studies covering sexual dysfunction, depression, nail-biting, study skills, weight control and smoking cessation. Overall, self-treatment outperformed control groups by 0.96 standard deviations. For independently assessed outcomes, the effect size was 0.47 standard deviations. Compared with treatments delivered by therapists, effects were higher by 0.07 standard deviations, though not significantly ($P > 0.05$), suggesting that self-care and assisted change approaches can be equally effective.

In the TTM, change is considered as an effortful process and not a discrete event, with readiness to change (in this case physical activity behaviour), described through five main stages. The first stage, Pre-contemplation, has at least two forms: the individual is either not thinking about change, or rejects the idea of changing. In the next stage, Contemplation, people are thinking seriously about changing in the near future. This is distinct from the third stage, Preparation, wherein the individual has started making infrequent changes. People who have made active change are in one of two further stages. Action describes when change is being undertaken regularly and frequently, but began only recently, and Maintenance is the stage when change has been regular and frequent for longer than six months.

Prochaska & DiClemente (1992) proposed that the essential elements of the TTM reflect over eighteen psychotherapeutic models, integrating over a hundred and forty treatment modalities. This shows the predominance of psychological factors within the model (Sallis & Owen 1999), which was developed to satisfy four main criteria (Prochaska & DiClemente 1994). These were to reflect both the diversity and essential unity of psychotherapy systems, to be empirically testable, to account for self-initiated and professionally assisted change across settings and behaviours, and to encourage therapists to learn from its elements and structure.

Freudenberg and colleagues (1995) listed principles for effective health promotions and these help to contextualize the widespread endorsement of TTM. These included tailoring interventions to the specific population and its setting, and involving participants in planning, implementation and evaluation. As part of this, efforts should be made to integrate individuals, social and physical environments, communities and policies. Three further criteria were offered: linking participants' concerns about health to broader life concerns and to a vision of a better society, using existing resources within the environment, and building on the strengths found among participants and their communities. Proponents of the TTM claim that these are all addressed in the model.

'Stages' also provides an alternative to the prevailing paradigm of 'Action'. Action-based approaches predicate (1) repeated interventions, (2) short-termism, and (3) a failure appropriately to invest in sustaining change and to deal with relapse. In the TTM, it is possible to determine positive change, whether or not people get into the action-based stages, or whether an intervention merely serves to support low levels of physical activity relapse. In this way, the TTM offers a framework for designing, delivering and evaluating intervention outcomes (Sarkin et al., 2001).

Most importantly within a health promotion context, not only does the TTM address self-change but also lends itself to the delivery of

Table 6.1   Motivational tasks associated with stage-matched progression

Stage of change	Motivational tasks
Precontemplation	Raise doubt about current situation or behaviour
Contemplation	Evoke powerful reasons for change and self-confidence to change
Preparation	Help determine the best way forward; try out some courses of action that feel 'comfortable'
Action	Help identify ways to support continued change
Maintenance	Help identify and enact strategies to prevent relapse

short, prescriptive (Dryden & Feltham, 1992) and client-centred counselling (Emmons & Rollnick, 2001) based on the individual's stage of change (see Table 6.1). Indeed, within counselling, readiness to change is not seen as something that individuals ought to do, or should want, it is the product of the interpersonal interactions between individuals and their helpers (Rollnick & Miller, 1995).

In physical activity terms, relapse is clearly a negative issue, since the physical benefits of participation are quickly lost. However, in the TTM, relapse is not a distinct stage but describes sustained withdrawal from being in Action or Maintenance (Velicer et al., 1990; Larimer, Larimer & Marlatt 1992; Marcus & Stanton, 1993). It remains conceptually problematic that relapse is inadequately differentiated from the more minor 'lapse' (Wing, 2000). Yet including Relapse as a sixth stage minimizes the stage differences found using the more conventional five-stage algorithm (Zhu & Ainsworth, 1999). By including Relapse as an option, individuals ticking this option may merely be indicating that they are in one of a range of inactive stages. Relapse is additionally characterized by features of Precontemplation, particularly where there is no intention of future involvement. Addressing intention represents an important refinement for stage devices (Jordan et al., 2002), and would also make classifications more conceptually consistent with the idea of change (Emmons & Rollnick, 2001).

Practitioners may be surprised at the on-going debates about stage definitions (e.g. Donovan et al., 1998; Reed, 1999). Yet these issues are important since inaccurate stage reporting prevents correctly identifying how interventions influence change and increases the chances of rejecting effective intervention approaches. Further, recent developments within the stage definitions show not only the diversity between stages, but also within stages. This suggests that identifying stage is only the first part of an overall process for optimizing the chances of producing change in individuals. This is well exemplified within the Contemplation stage (see later).

Each stage, as the first of three central constructs within the TTM (the others being processes of change and levels of change), is now considered in more detail, beginning with the least active stages. As highlighted earlier, whilst research on models, including the TTM, and physical activity behaviour change in young people is limited, where possible, evidence is presented from studies with young people and younger populations (e.g. college students).

TTM: the Contemplation stage

The Contemplation stage here is used to characterize one of the inactive stages. A number of studies have identified contemplators' key processes within cognitive, rational-emotive and cognitive behavioural approaches (Miller & Rollnick, 1991), and some studies have focused on exercise behaviour (Marcus et al., 1992; 2000). A number of studies have shown that counsellors can help individuals to increase their use (e.g. Dunn et al., 1997) and so, it is expected, increase the likelihood of their becoming more active.

However, working with and influencing contemplators may be problematic. For example, stage-specific exercise preferences (n = 2600 students; Naylor & McKenna, 1995) and stage-specific barriers (n = 182 adults; Eves, Mant & Clarke, 1996, and employees; Heesch, Brown & Blanton, 1999) are relatively common. Further, recent quantitative analyses have identified three subtypes within Contemplation, each with a different capacity for change (Gorely & Bruce, 2000). These are no change, wanting to change, and ready to change, and they confirm that the change needs of exercise contemplators are not fully understood. It is important to understand that cross-sectional data do little to characterize change efforts in the different stages, and there is a need for both qualitative and longitudinal evidence to address these shortfalls.

Prochaska, Norcross & DiClemente, (1996) identified that contemplators may use four 'delay tactics': searching for absolute certainty, waiting for the magic moment, wishful thinking and premature action. Premature action is a delay tactic because action cannot be supported and so relapses, creating further delay. In a recent qualitative study, McKenna & Francis (2003) showed how 'chronic' contemplators (confirmed as being in contemplation for at least three months) can display low motivation, apathy or even antagonism toward physical activity advice. Despite being interested in changing in the future, contemplators' language and demeanour suggest ambivalence and/or resistance to changing. This issue is highly significant since the counselling literature consistently emphasizes the importance of the interaction between clients and supporters (Garfield 1994; Rollnick & Miller 1995; Emmons & Rollnick 2001).

TTM: the Maintenance stage

In the Maintenance stage, different levels of effort may be required to support physical activity behaviour (Cardinal & Levy 1999; Wing 2000). Yet, within the TTM, Maintenance is considered as the stage of effortful but sustained change. The concept of allostasis (McEwan & Stellar, 1993) may more accurately represent living as a physical activity maintainer, since it describes change in the presence of ongoing demands. This concept is especially useful for distinguishing sustained change from the concept of effortless action (or habit), which may be termed 'termination'. Termination is associated with 100 per cent confidence for continuing with this behavioural pattern (Cardinal & Levy, 1999) and is clearly relevant to the original model, which focused on cessation behaviours. However, in the context of modern living environments that encourage sedentary living, this has to be a doubtful proposition for many people. Surprisingly though, given current concerns for levels of physical inactivity, maintainers are often the largest single stage. In young people, they have been reported to comprise 31.1 per cent of 937 college students (Silver-Wallace et al., 2000) and 49.3 per cent of 819 US adolescents (Nigg & Courneya, 1998).

In adults, although more than six in ten exercise maintainers remained in this stage over six months (Plotnikoff et al., 2001), there may be a belief that they have no exercise problems or barriers, and so need no support. Yet this may vary across physical activity behaviours. For example, in interviews with experienced regular and frequent participants, commuter cycling was a fragile behaviour, given that it routinely involved dangerous or negative daily experiences (McKenna & Whatley, in press). Similarly, of 133 working women who self-reported being in maintenance, 41.7 per cent felt that lack of time, due to work demands, was a barrier to their physical activity behaviour. Time is also frequently cited as a barrier to exercise by young people (see later). Further, 'lack of discipline' was endorsed by 41.7 per cent of maintainers. These features underline the need for support processes to be enacted for even the active population.

Failing to support maintainers may be as unethical as failing to promote behaviour change in individuals who are not yet ready to change (Whitehead, 1997; Bunton et al., 2000), as maintainers need support to develop relapse-prevention skills (Larimer & Marlatt 1992; Rothman 2000). Supporting these specific skills may be a problem for many professionals. In one cross-sectional UK survey (Aznar & McKenna, 1996), 48 per cent of practice nurses felt effective in promoting physical activity with 'all' or 'most' precontemplators, but this fell to 8 per cent with maintainers. Indeed, health and other professionals may recognise that their competence varies for supporting the needs of individuals in the different stages. The next TTM concept, processes of change, helps to illustrate how individuals are different across the stages.

TTM: processes of change

Importantly, as well as describing stages of readiness to change, the TTM integrates processes, or strategies, of change (see Table 6.2). Based on the ten most common processes, statistical relationships confirm that cognitive (or experiential) processes are used to progress from the early stages, while behavioural processes support being in the active stages of change. A particular feature of the TTM is that the processes of change reflect perceptions of the environment and their influence on behavioural decision-making.

The Processes of Exercise Questionnaire (PCQ) (Marcus et al., 1992) comprises 40 items which reduce to 10 subscales for each of the major processes. Mean scores for how often each process is used are calculated (T-scores are used to provide standardized scores when subscales have an unequal number of contributing items) and then plotted. The resulting line graph, with stage on the horizontal axis, has been described as drawing a 'mountain profile' with low levels of use depicted in the inactive stages, rising for the active stages. It is important to keep in mind that these graphs do not depict individuals who are themselves changing; they can give the misleading impression that stage-change is consistently associated with increased use of the different processes.

Table 6.2 Processes of change, their theoretical origins and how they are operationalized

Process	Goals
Experiential	
Consciousness-raising	Increasing information about self and problem and potential solutions
Dramatic relief	Experiencing and expressing feelings about one's problems and solutions; intense emotional reactions to current behaviours
Self re-evaluation	Changing assessment of feelings and thoughts about self and problem
Social liberation	Creating increased social alternatives for behaviours that are not problematic
Social re-evaluation	Changing appraisal of how problem affects others
Behavioural	
Self-liberation	Choosing and committing to act, or belief in ability to change
Counter-conditioning	Changing reactions to stimuli; substituting alternatives for problem behaviours
Stimulus control	Avoiding stimuli that elicit problem behaviours; changing environments
Helping relationships	Enlisting help for change from someone who cares
Reinforcement management	Changing reinforcers and contingencies for a new behaviour; rewarding self, or being rewarded by others, for making changes

Source: After Prochaska & DiClemente (1992) and Prochaska, Norcross & DiClemente (1996).

However, there are some problems with the processes of change. Given the need for predictive outcomes, it is problematic that a questionnaire measuring processes of change predicted only 14 per cent of variance in self-reported exercise (Engel et al., 1999). In another study, the same questionnaire only contributed to explaining 15 per cent variance in daily energy expenditure (Plotnikoff et al., 1999). In the PACE project (Calfas et al., 1997), all psychosocial variables, including the experimental design, explained only 34 per cent of changes in physical activity behaviour.

Furthermore, a recent one-year exercise study empirically confirmed only one of eight process-based hypotheses (Plotnikoff et al., 2001). These data suggest that the 'processes of change' may be inadequately conceptualized for exercise, meaning that even state-of-the art physical activity promotions based on this theory may be misdirected and fail to address the no-change experience of many sedentary individuals.

TTM: levels of change

Levels of change reflect where individuals perceive the control lies for their potential to change. Five levels are proposed:

1 situational (e.g. barriers such as time, mental energy, living arrangements)
2 cognitive (e.g. perceptions, attitudes, beliefs)
3 interpersonal (e.g. potential conflict with significant others)
4 family systems (e.g. potential conflict with family values)
5 intrapersonal (e.g. potential conflict with strong and fundamental personal values) (Prochaska, Norcross & DiClemente, 1996).

The low level of study relating to levels of change, however, is surprising. Counselling based on the levels is typically achieved on a one-to-one basis since it focuses on first dealing with the strongest barriers. Different schools adopt different approaches and these define the 'school', though most of the integrated models within the TTM are best validated for the levels closest to number one. Shorter interventions are deemed to be more suited to the levels with a number closer to one, which itself indicates lower resistance to, and probability of, change (Ratner & Yandoli, 1996). It is proposed that where the individual perceives the controlling system 'situational' then change may be considered more probable. On the other hand, where control is perceived to be 'intrapersonal', it is impeded by inner conflicts, making short-term change improbable. The likelihood of change occurring is also likely to hinge on the skills of the deliverer.

Notwithstanding the problems of the TTM, the model appeals to health and physical activity promoters because it expresses an easily understandable and systematic relationship between the stages and processes of change. This is further supplemented by its systematic relationship with two other dominant theoretical perspectives: decision balance (Janis & Mann, 1977) and self-efficacy (Bandura, 1977; 1986; 1997). For these reasons, interest in the model stems from its claim to be a, perhaps the, generic model which subsumes the other elements of theory.

TTM: Decision Balance

The Decision Balance (DB) construct relates to the ways in which individuals make decisions in their daily lives (Janis & Mann, 1977). This is based on two themes: the benefits of changing (the Pros) and the disadvantages of changing (the Cons), and how they balance. Within cross-sectional studies of physical activity, the balance of scores between questionnaire responses illustrates that the Pros overtake the Cons in the Preparation stage (Prochaska, 1994). DB scores are also consistent with self-reported physical activity, suggesting their concurrent validity. Scores of 673 university students recruited to a physical activity intervention (Naylor & McKenna, 1995) matched those found in free-living adults. For the students, total physical activity scores differed in line with stage of change.

The components of the 16-item DB scale for physical activity (Marcus et al., 1992) includes nine Pros and seven Cons. The many such self-efficacy scales often address common themes, including tiredness or lacking energy and having no time for family and friends. These themes have also been explored in large-scale national studies, such as the Allied Dunbar National Fitness Survey (ADNFS) (Sports Council & Health Education Authority, 1992). Within this UK study, barriers to physical activity were explored in over three thousand adults. Based on 'applies to me/doesn't apply to me' responses, almost 20 per cent of 16–25-year-olds endorsed ' I am not the sporty type', and 45.8 per cent endorsed the barrier 'have not got the time'. This former figure has received extensive attention. More recent UK evidence shows that among 420 respondents aged 16–24 years, the most endorsed of five barriers are lack of leisure time (57.7 per cent), followed by lack of money (49.0 per cent) and lack of motivation (48.7 per cent) (Chinn et al., 1999).

While the presence of individual barriers can be important, the whole issue of the constraining effects of barriers requires closer consideration. For example, within the ADNFS a total of 18 potential barriers could be reported, yet among 16–25-year-olds, 100 (of 651) reported having no physical activity barriers and 353 reported three or fewer. While it may be expected that numerous barriers may impair self-efficacy for physical activity (Jaffee et al., 1999), this may not be automatic. Individuals who regularly remind themselves of the negative effects of these factors may profit from process-related counselling, which focuses on how individuals perceive their environment. Intervention studies confirm that more frequent positive thoughts of this type predict positive change attempts.

The ADNFS also addressed positive values for involvement in physical activity. In DB terms, these have strong links to the Pros of changing. Here younger respondents (n=558) reported no values for involvement in regular vigorous activity that exceeded those of over-25-year-olds (n=3132). In contrast, older adults consistently reported having stronger beliefs that this level of physical activity would (1) be fun, (2) improve one's social life, (3) improve physical appearance and (4) improve mental functioning. However, Eves, Mant & Clarke (1996) cautioned against the widespread endorsement of motives like 'fun' to encourage inactive individuals. They argue that this may only be relevant to those who see physical activity as something for people 'like themselves', or for people who are already active.

In active US working women (Jaffee et al., 1999), the most endorsed of 15 motives were (1) improved cardiovascular fitness, (2) improved muscle tone and (3) on-going good health. Fahrenwald & Walker (2003) showed that the Pros for physical activity among young mothers included increased strength, stress relief and getting back into shape having been pregnant. In contrast, the Cons included bad weather, child care and fatigue. Jordan and colleagues (2002) added further Cons in studying 223 undergraduates, including 'my family and friends have to wait for me to shower', and 'I would feel selfish if I exercised regularly'. These suggest that affective elements are implicated in the Cons for exercising. These features are likely to combine in unique ways, which endorses the use of the DB worksheet for individual interventions, which might help link to the levels of change (see earlier).

A major strength of the DB approach is that it helps to prevent isolating physical activity from its 'real-life' competitors such as TV viewing or being with inactive friends. This helps individuals to generate a more realistic perspective about 'exercise in my life', as opposed to generic statements about attitudes or values associated with physical activity. It also helps practitioners and others to develop a realistic grasp of the likelihood of an individual to change. This is not always positive towards physical activity.

In some cases, particular features of the physical activity mode may represent an insurmountable barrier in their current context. For example, the widespread decline in active commuting to school through cycling may have resulted from the overall DB. The Cons here are likely to include exposure to especially busy intersections, need for safety equipment, exposure to pollution, risk of cycle theft, and lack of parental supervision. Placed against the possible Pros, ready access of cycling, and health and fitness outcomes, it is clear how parents might prefer the 'school run', or some other form of motorized transport. Yet individuals who hold these views about cycling may describe a markedly different DB for cycling while on holiday in a different community, suggesting the importance of regularly revising individual's DB.

Critique of the TTM

While a specific critique of the different elements of the TTM has already been offered, there remains a need for a general commentary about the overall appeal of the model. Despite its popularity with practitioners, theoreticians like Bandura (1997) have been especially critical of the proposition that stages of change are discrete. Taking the view that human functioning is too complex and multifaceted to be categorized into a few distinct stages, he suggested the possibility that stage concept may be redundant in the context of current theorizing.

There is a need to develop moderate intensity physical activity formulations in scales so they match the high test-rest reliabilities for vigorous intensity physical activity found among US and Australian students (Leslie et al., 2003). In addition, there are ethical concerns about some of the delivery issues proposed within the model. For example, there has been debate about the ethics of not recommending action when an individual is in a preactive stage (Whitehead, 1997). Equally, there is a need to systematically address the downside of regular physical activity involvement to reduce rates of injury.

Finally, beyond physical activity, there have been critical evaluations which question whether the model applies to all behavioural arenas (Ashworth, 1997; Bandura, 1997) and whether stage-matching is as specific as is suggested by the theory (Weinstein, Rothman & Sutton, 1998). The assumption of generic quality and applicability makes the application of the TTM to physical activity scenarios highly appealing, notwithstanding ongoing debates about whether the model is transtheoretical or atheoretical.

Self-efficacy and the Social Cognitive Theory

Although in its own right the Social Cognitive Theory (SCT) may be seen as a competence-based theory, and has commanded extensive research interest (Biddle & Nigg, 2000), it has also been integrated within the TTM. However, recent studies have shown that the SCT is central to the study of change (Nigg & Courneya, 1998), which justifies considering it in its own right.

Social Cognitive Theory (SCT) (Bandura, 1986; 1997) is a general psychological theory based on the idea that human behaviour is guided by the ability to consider future consequences of a given behaviour, and the ability to form perceptions about one's own capabilities to perform a behaviour. In particular, the model addresses behavioural determinants of the person, the environment and features of the physical activity behaviour being considered (Silver-Wallace et al., 2000). Within SCT, self-efficacy, outcome expectations and self-evaluated dissatisfaction are assumed to be important mediators of behaviour and behaviour change. Self-efficacy is a central feature of the theory (Bandura, 1986; 1997) and is a person's belief that they can accomplish some task. It is hypothesized to be the most important component influencing choice, effort and persistence. Outcome expectancies are a person's expectation that a given behaviour will lead to a given outcome. In other words, they describe the expected consequences of successful involvement in physical activity. The difference between outcome expectations and self-efficacy is that a person may believe that a given behaviour results in a desired outcome, but not believe that they can perform the given behaviour. Self-dissatisfaction reflects how an individual compares his or her performance or behaviour to a standard and reacts with satisfaction or dissatisfaction. Dissatisfaction may lead to a change in behaviour, whereas satisfaction with a behaviour but a desire to avoid dissatisfaction in the future may lead to continuation of a behaviour.

Within physical activity studies, self-efficacy has been operationalized to reflect the specific expectancies (or self-confidences) to overcome the day-to-day barriers of being tired, in a bad mood, dealing with bad weather or having no time (e.g. Marcus et al., 1992). Nigg and Courneya (1998, p. 217) added extra items to address the particular life experiences of the young people in their Canadian study: 'I am confident I can exercise regularly when I have homework to do...when friends call me to go out...when there is a good show on TV...when I am on my own.'

Cross-sectional studies have shown that physical activity self-efficacy scores tend to be higher across stages of change, with the highest scores found in Maintenance and the lowest in Precontemplation (e.g. Naylor & McKenna, 1995). Consistent patterns of scores were found in a study of UK students (Naylor & McKenna, 1995). Further, findings from this study converged with others showing that males at each stage consistently report higher self-efficacy scores than females ($P < 0.05$).

However, there is an important but unexpected feature associated with two recent intervention studies. Surprisingly, both studies were associated with reductions in self-efficacy (Kerr & McKenna, 2000; Hillsdon et al., 2001). The first was a one-week, work-based intervention, while the second was a nationwide UK physical activity promotion. It may be that raising awareness of physical activity may underline to respondents the extent of change they would need to make in order for physical activity to become a reality. Taking a lead from literature about the effects of interventions based on fear appeals here (Witte & Allen, 2000) and it may be that 'positive message' physical activity interventions will have their greatest impact when messages are accompanied by advice about the appropriate responsive actions.

The Theory of Reasoned Action and the Theory of Planned Behaviour

The Theory of Reasoned Action (TRA) and the Theory of Planned Behaviour (TPB) have a long history within studies of health-related behaviours, including physical activity, exercise and sports behaviour. The TRA (Fishbein & Ajzen, 1975) and the TPB (Ajzen, 1991) are general models concerned with the relationships between attitudes and volitional behaviour. The basic premise is that intention, the plan to carry out a behaviour, is the most important determinant of behaviour. In the TRA, intention to undertake a behaviour is associated with conceptually distinctive, but belief-based, elements. These elements are arranged in three layers: (1) 'attitude' towards the new behaviour and (2) 'normative beliefs' (or subjective norms) for this behaviour form the first layer. The individual and combined actions of these variables create the second layer in the model – 'intention'. Intention is then linked to the final layer of 'behaviour'. Attitude is a function of an individual's beliefs that a behaviour will lead to a certain outcome and an evaluation of whether this outcome is important and would be worthwhile. Subjective norm is based on an individual's beliefs about significant others' opinions regarding the behaviour, and a motivation to comply with the expectations of others. The TRA was, however, criticized for assuming that all behaviours were under the same degree of individual control. Thus, the TPB is a development of the TRA (Ajzen & Fishbein, 1970) which addresses this criticism and extends the model to include the concept of perceived behavioural control (PBC) within the first layer. PBC, defined as 'the perceived ease or difficulty of performing the behaviour' (Ajzen, 1988, p. 132) reflects the extent to which individuals perceive they have control over external and internal factors that may interfere with performing a behaviour. PBC is determined by a control belief (personal beliefs about resources and opportunities to perform a given behaviour), and perceived power to control the factors that facilitate or inhibit behaviour. Thus, 'control' is modelled as interplaying with 'attitude', 'intention', and potentially 'behaviour'.

A contemporary concern is to explore specific exercise belief predictors (Rosen, 2000). Not surprisingly, these beliefs influenced exercise behaviour among fitness club members in Greece (Theodorakis, 1994). Similarly, in young US mothers, believing that exercise increased strength, represented a sense of accomplishment, offered stress relief or helped them to get back into shape after being pregnant all supported more regular activity involvement (Fahrenwald & Walker, 2003).

Beliefs may also help to explain sedentary lifestyles, although 'normative beliefs' have an inconsistent track record for physical activity behaviour. Steptoe and colleagues (1997) examined physical activity behaviours and beliefs of over sixteen thousand students from 21 European countries and found that even within a single country such as the UK, beliefs had a different predictive effect. Odds ratios were calculated to predict exercise behaviour based on responses to a one-to-ten scale measuring the belief in 'the importance of regular exercise for health'. For English students, each increment increased the predictive value for exercising regularly by a factor of five (OR = 5.54), whereas for Scottish students the predictive value was over three times stronger (OR = 18.25).

If negative beliefs are predictive of sedentary living, it is worrying that in a representative UK survey of adults (n = 1971), as age increased so did the proportion of respondents reporting being 'not really an active person' (Capibas, 1999). However, the relationship of positive beliefs with positive behaviours is not always consistent. Of 730 lapsed fitness club members, over six in ten believed that their membership was a positive experience (Fitness Industry Association, 2000), while in older Canadian women normative beliefs predicted exercise intention (Wankel & Mummery, 1993).

There may be merit in considering how negative beliefs contribute to negative physical activity behaviour. It is not clear how beliefs predict behaviours such as active commuting to school or work, neither is it clear how beliefs support unhealthy behaviours within physical activity. This may include different norms for pedestrian violations (Diaz, 2002), avoiding wearing cycling helmets (Bergman et al., 1990; Quine, Rutter & Arnold, 2001), or not wearing safety equipment while competing in contact sports (Finch, McIntosh & McCrory, 2001).

However, the theory is not without its proponents for change or development. Ajzen (1991) proposed the need to explore not only how often behaviours occur, but also how often more powerful beliefs are enacted. Others, such as Chatzisarantis et al., (in press), propose the need to consider further themes within the model, especially the role of perceived autonomy support (where significant others encourage decision-making while offering minimal pressure and high support for personal preferences; people who are autonomy-supportive will restrict their use of 'should', 'must' and 'ought' with regard to physical activity behaviour in others) and previous physical activity history. There is also a need to address how the contributory elements perform within the changes of adoption–relapse cycles of physical activity behaviour. Others note that subjective norms do not necessarily capture the full extent of social influence, a point that is addressed in the subsequent section of this chapter. Finally, it remains a problem that researchers operationalize the constructs differently (Quine, Rutter & Arnold, 2001), making their conversion to practical intervention approaches more challenging.

Social approaches

Just as diseases are subject to a social gradient (Syme, 2000), so too are physical activity patterns linked to socio-economic status (Sports Council & Health Education Authority, 1992; Lee & Cubbin, 2002). Social approaches are addressed within this chapter for a simple reason: lifestyle factors only influence about 50 per cent of disease variance (Davison, Frankl & Davey Smith, 1992), while social factors such as 'control' flatten the established social gradient for disease (Marmot et al., 1997). Further, while most models of behaviour change explain less than 40 per cent of variance (Spence & Lee, 2003), social factors, such as connectedness, have relative risk factors for reducing coronary heart disease (2.3 to 2.8) at least equivalent to that of smoking (2.2) (Berkman, 2000) and sedentary living (1.9). In this section, the term 'social paradigm' is used to encompass a range of concepts prefixed by social, including inclusion, network, capital, cohesion, connection and support, and the health-promotion terms of 'population' and 'community' (Merzel & D'Afflitti, 2003).

Firstly, although a social approach can offer distinctive features and practices, some social elements share common ground with the psychological models addressed in the previous section. For example, Table 6.2 describes the process of helping relationships, which have close associations with features in social support – in a social perspective, support can be seen as a feature of personal networks. Within the SCT (see earlier), the self-efficacy to say 'no' to friends or family is another feature of the social experience. Finally, being clear on the social consequences of saying 'no' to friends, in spite of the social consequences, has close association with DB theory addressed earlier. This final example begins to come close to the approach offered by a distinctive sociological, or social policy, approach. However, within the social paradigm the relevance of these concepts is questioned until they are made relevant to the lived experiences of individuals (Bryman, 1988).

Consistent with the idea of stage-matching suggested by the TTM, social approaches to physical activity promotion are concerned with developing and delivering 'appropriate' and 'relevant' programmes. In the social paradigm, these themes are determined by factors like values. However, unlike psychologically based models, they do not prescribe specific practice, but instead offer principles for developing programmes.

Social models formulate ways of developing this practice, the embodiment of which is reflexivity (Caplan, 1993). Reflexivity has a high position within the social paradigm because all health (and physical activity) promotion decisions are rooted in politically-related decision-making (Seedhouse, 1997), and all such knowledge is socially constructed (Kerlinger, 1986). To be reflexive, physical activity promoters will consider why they value particular forms of evidence over others (e.g. 'accepting' the evidence from randomized controlled trials but 'rejecting' in-depth qualitative studies of physical activity behaviour), why programmes are considered suitable in a given setting or community and how they will work. One further essential difference that exists between psychological and social-based approaches is the willingness of physical activity professionals, who are often trained in psychological models, to learn from local individuals about local working practices and politics (Syme, 2000). In effect, working in a 'social' way requires foregoing the status of 'expert'.

The following activities illustrate these ideas. These exercises are borrowed from Raphael (2000) and reworked for relevance to physical activity promotion.

Activity

Page 147 shows different purposes for promoting physical activity. Responses capitalize on different understandings of how physical activity contributes to 'health'. Which do you endorse and why?

Physical activity promotion is about improving medical treatment.
Physical activity promotion is about changing lifestyles.
Physical activity promotion is about helping people to cope with their social conditions.
Physical activity promotion is about changing social conditions.

Activity

The second activity shows how physical activity promotions can begin from political understandings. Consider the sets of propositions. Which do you endorse? Give your reasons.

Environments cause inactivity	OR	Motivation causes inactivity
Inactivity causes CHD	OR	Misunderstanding of physical activity causes CHD
Poor people have inactive lifestyles	OR	Neighbourhoods cause inactivity

Without being overly prescriptive, it is suggested that strong endorsement of the first option in each pair suggests a social understanding of why physical activity might be promoted. Endorsing the second option suggests a preference for more individualized interventions.

Consistent with the idea of matching proposed by the TTM, Cohen & Herbert (1996) have shown the value in matching social support to individuals' pre-existing social patterns. This helps to widen programme appeal. Given that group-based physical activity is likely to serve any of the five main purposes for being in a group (belonging, intimacy, growth, stability and generativity), then it is clear that there is scope for refining delivery to meet social needs. Further, this suggests that responsiveness to a programme can be matched not only for stage of change, but also for social needs. Indeed, as many social factors as motivational 'barriers' are likely to be present before beginning any physical activity programme. This list might include factors such as residential and employment instability, financial vulnerability, low educational attainment, low social trust, few social connections and limited experience of group-based activities. These features characterize low levels of 'social capital' (Putnam, 2000).

Another reason for the relative inattention to social elements is that these processes are complex, if not intractable, and are not necessarily within the control of individuals, researchers or practitioners. Hillman, Adams & Whitelegg (1991), for example, showed that the parental 'licence' offered to 9-year-olds in 1979, was only available to 13-year-olds by 1991. In the same period, 80 per cent of 7–8-year-olds went to school on their own in the 1970s, which fell to fewer than one in ten in 1990.

Key social issues that may have relevance to models of physical activity behaviour (and intervention) include explaining the social processes that underpin sedentary individuals who actively prevent family, friends or acquaintances from becoming more active (e.g. Jordan et al., 2002; McKenna & Francis, 2003). Social processes may also help to address why particular groups are resistant to physical activity promotions, or 'drop out' from existing programmes, as is common amongst adolescent females (Riddoch, 1998). At least part of the reason for groups being 'hard to reach' may involve social explanations and, given that social processes often involve interaction, this suggests that problems may exist on both sides of the interaction with promoters. Although some behaviours are obviously inactive, such as playing computer games or the school run, they also have a hidden but profoundly negative community consequence (e.g. restrict involvement in community affairs/interactions).

Two examples are presented of how physical activity promoters might respond to a given programme outcome. The first underlines how thinking derived from the medical model may influence the thinking about cause and effect. The second shows the common ground between 'social' physical activity promoters and those who prefer medical-model perspectives. Both examples have implications for the working relationships with any group.

Scenario

A 3-month physical activity intervention is delivered in an area with high health needs. Adherence is high and the programme considered a success. However, when the external support is removed, a high level of drop-out occurs. Why did this happen?

Explanations using medical model of thinking

Explanation 1: It is due to some 'lack' in these individuals.

Attribution theory describes how we explain a cause and effect and is sometimes referred to as the psychology of the 'good guys' (Hewstone, 1989). Success is due to 'internal' factors of effort and strategy, while 'external' explanations (luck, chance) are seen as excuses, with all the associations of bias, stigmatization and blame that may follow.

Explanation 2: The right programme, the wrong place.

Social features not only influence behaviour, but also beliefs, attitudes and social norms for risk (see TRA/TPB earlier). These can be different to, or possibly conflict with, those that health/physical activity promoters derive from the medical model and which support programme delivery. Summarizing these issues, and underlining how promoting 'physical activity-as-healthy-lifestyle' may be a problematic message in some neighbourhoods, Davison, Frankl & Davey Smith (1992) note how three interlocking fields of influence featured in lifestyle narratives of Welsh adults. Not surprisingly, these included personal differences, social environment and physical environment. However, a further field was also noted, that of 'non-control' (which they distinguish from the value-laden term, 'fatalistic'). Shinn & Toohey (2003) suggest that such explanations may describe a tendency to underestimate the real power of their environments, which they term 'context minimisation error'.

At another level, social exclusion can result in a negative underlying physiology, resulting from denied social access. These denials may affect contact with friends or family, community services and physical locations, and are associated with a poorer health status in a range of indices.

Recent evidence from participants in a community walking programme in a low income district of Perth, Western Australia, confirmed that social capital was enhanced through the programme (Bayly & Bull, 2001). These benefits may appear unfamiliar to medical-model proponents, but they show how the social paradigm offers alternative, and perhaps more realizable, outcomes in some communities. Often these features are seen as important processes, but are overlooked as important intervention outcomes. They included building social networks, developing trust between individuals and organizations, feeling connected, tolerating diversity and helping others within and beyond the walking group. A new scale, first used in the 2001 Health Survey for England, is now available to measure key markers of social capital and social exclusion (Bajekal & Purdon, 2001).

The social changes described in this walking group may also affect individual biochemistry. Plausible evidence suggests that neuroendocrine and behavioural features of numerous disease states reflect acute and chronic social experience. This includes depressive and anxiety disorders (Kiecolt-Glaser et al., 1988; 2002) and coronary heart disease (Krantz &

McCeney, 2002). Some of these pathological processes can originate in adolescence (Kuh & Ben-Shlomo, 1997) and may be initiated through negative social experiences (Repetti, McGrath & Ishikawa, 1996). Some even have a 'lag' that only becomes manifest in middle age (e.g. Siegler et al., 1992). It remains to be seen how physical activity may influence these different processes, and in how many people, though there is a clear case for accepting that an individual's social experience has powerful health effects.

However, while we have focused on positive elements of the social paradigm, critical perspectives also require attention. For example, Doyal (2003) has highlighted how health can be 'gendered'. Extending her arguments to physical activity promotion, it is possible to see how gender-based 'cultural devaluation' can begin even at an early age. Unwillingness to correspond to social norms may create physical activity disadvantages for young people. The pejorative label of 'not being manly enough' to cope with rough (or dangerous) play or 'being like a girl' if interested in dance activities may do untold damage to the physical activity potential of some adolescent males. These issues reflect 'social' perspectives of masculinity. Equally, 'sex'-based perspectives which relate to biology, may just as profoundly disadvantage females. In this context, the beneficial effects of physical activity on bone-building and the concerns for developing reproductive functioning obviously cross the social and medical realms.

For other groups, social 'differences' may create problems in generating a productive dialogue across ethnic groups (Gunaratnam, 2003). Other social approaches focus on the characteristics that unite groups, including cultural and ethnic targeting. However, despite the attempts to provide a working framework for cultural health promotion (e.g. Kreuter et al., 2003), even well-intentioned approaches can miss essential features of the social norms for ethnic groups (Kumanyika, 2003). Further, even within these populations there can be immense diversity leading to the need for unique approaches.

Settings as social factors

Locations provide another element of the social paradigm. Sociologists emphasize that 'space' offers the chance to consider how social constructions of behaviour develop and circulate. Reflecting many qualitative perspectives, authors like Bourdieu (1977) and Giddens (1984) use labels such as 'locale', 'locality', or 'habitus' to illustrate the 'felt value' of particular locations. The 115 'No ball games' signs found in a single

UK housing estate (Children's Society and Play Council, 2003) may be as restrictive to play as are perceptions of particular spaces (that individuals might never enter) for active travel/commuting. The felt value of a setting is filtered by individual needs for autonomy, self-development, intimacy, choice and control. These produce powerful behavioural forces, which in physical activity terms contribute to the appeal of different forms of physical activity, from individual to group-based sessions.

Physical activity promoters also consider location when planning where to deliver their services or interventions. Based on considerations of access, responsiveness and equity, to name but a few, favoured venues seem to be schools and colleges, worksites and general practices. Physical activity promotion in schools is addressed in Chapters 7 and 10 of this text.

General practice approaches

It is unclear what proportion of general practitioners (GPs) regularly promote specific forms of physical activity, although it is known that of 1232 inactive Australians, 38 per cent identified their doctor as a preferred source of exercise information and support (Booth et al., 1997). This figure was lowest, however, in younger people (aged 18–39) (one in five) and highest in people aged 60+ (one in two). Young people may have other preferred settings for physical activity promotions (e.g. school, community) or uses for medical consultations, and/or they may find that contemporary delivery is unappealing to them.

The idea of promoting health in young people within primary care has a mixed history, reflecting the balance between their preferences and the willingness of staff to approach them. A recent review (Walker & Townsend, 1999) confirmed that general practice staff rarely offered advice to teenagers and offered even less physical activity support. Practice nurses consider adolescents to be a difficult group (Bekaert, 2003), suggesting that their needs are unlikely to be addressed. Young people consistently report concerns about confidentiality of general-practice-based interventions (Walker & Townsend, 1999). However, in one of the few general-practice-based health promotion controlled trials, Walker et al. (2002) found positive exercise effects among 14–15-year-olds over three months. In the absence of a substantial evidence base for young people, exploring the issues within adults may highlight physical activity possibilities.

Motivational Interviewing (MI) (Rollnick & Miller, 1995; Emmons & Rollnick 2001) is one counselling style especially suited to medical settings such as general practice. MI has many themes that are consistent with the TTM, although there are important distinctions that question the appropriateness of using client-centred approaches to approach groups (Rollnick & Miller, 1995), as 'stages' might suggest. These issues centre on where the 'power' lies within consultations. Within MI the individual is the expert, since the purpose of the professional is to help facilitate a desire for change. This clearly presents a possible problem where physical activity specialists contribute to health/ physical activity promotions. Their skills centre on physical activity, whereas this may not figure in the individual's perspective of needs. In the social paradigm, the aim is for individuals to develop their own agendas for change.

Canadian research has confirmed that fewer than one in twelve doctors felt that evidence for exercise effects was an important barrier to their promotional efforts (Kennedy & Meeuwisse, 2003). Rather, their needs may centre on developing approaches that 'fit' within daily practice schedules. TTM-derived interventions can make physical activity promotions more systematic and client-centred. The 'A' factor approach has a similar theoretical background (Pinto, Goldstein & Mascus, 1998; Chapman, Adam & Stockford, 2001; Rosal et al., 2001) and offers a further intervention style for physical activity promotion. Here GPs use different 'A' factors (e.g. ask, assess, advise, assure, arrange a follow-up, and applaud) to promote physical activity. Critically, patients remember when their GPs use the 'A' factors. With appropriate training, 83 per cent of doctors talked about exercise in consultations and 99 per cent of patients recalled being counselled (Albright et al., 2000).

One recent study has integrated both the stages and the 'A' factor approach (McKenna & Vernon, in press). Responding to a questionnaire, 234 GPs described how they used 'A' factors with patients in the stages of change. The resulting ORs (odds ratios) indicate the predictive value of endorsing using the different 'A' factors for regularly promoting physical activity. GPs who reported arranging follow-up meetings with pre-contemplator patients were almost five times more likely to report also promoting physical activity regularly with their patients (OR = 4.93). Passing contemplators on to a GP referral scheme achieved an odds ratio of 2.34, while the value for asking relapsed patients about their lifestyle physical activity was 2.61. The findings not only suggest that the concept of stage-matching is relevant to GP promotion of physical activity, but also the value of these particular practices in developing locally-based training.

Conclusions

Perhaps one of the strongest reasons why the TTM is often preferred over other approaches is that it offers a range of intervention options. This complements most practitioners' preference for innovation and creativity over evidence. However, a considerably strengthened evidence base is needed to support this approach over others if the model is to continue to receive the support it currently enjoys. A central feature in building such an evidence base is the need to explore which elements of the different models are associated with behaviour changes within interventions.

It remains an issue that many of the models that guide physical activity promotion interventions are based on change alone. This may not seem an altogether bad thing, yet it is also essential to understand how interventions can produce change when they borrow ideas and practices from the models of change. This places a high priority on the need for what MacDonald & Green (2001, p. 244) call the 'theory of the intervention'.

There is a need to compare strong theoretically-derived interventions, particularly with young people, and at the same time to pay careful attention to treatment fidelity to overcome the tendency of practitioners and others to 'want to do the best' for young people. These studies are likely to be large and perhaps even multinational, and will require extensive funding to ensure the rigour that is required. This will help to contribute to the evidence base which is currently slim. Once this is established, the challenge of applying and making it relevant to professional practice must be faced.

Discussion point   As is evident from this chapter, theoretical models (e.g. TTM, SCT, TRA/TPB) tend to have been used primarily with adults and by health practitioners (e.g. health and physical activity promotion specialists).

Why do you think this is?

How might such models be usefully employed with young people and by others involved in working with young people (e.g. physical education teachers, exercise instructors/leaders) to influence their physical activity behaviour?

References

Ajzen, I. (1988) *Attitudes, Personality and Behaviour*. Milton Keynes: Open University.
Ajzen, I. (1991) The theory of planned behavior, *Organizational Behavior and Human Decision Processes*, **50**, 179–211.

Ajzen, I. & Fishbein, M. (1970) The prediction of behaviour from attitudinal and normative beliefs, *Journal of Personality and Social Psychology*, **6**, 466–87.

Albright, C. L., Cohen, S., Gibbons, L., Miller, B, Sallis, J. F., Imai, K. et al. (2000) Incorporating physical activity advice into primary care: physician-delivered advice within the Activity Counseling Trial, *American Journal of Preventive Medicine*, **18**, 225–34.

Ashworth, P. (1997) Breakthrough or bandwagon? Are interventions tailored to stage of change more effective than non-staged interventions? *Health Education Journal*, **56**, 166–74.

Aznar, S. & McKenna, J. (1996) Coronary heart disease risk reduction: how effective do nurses think they are in changing patients' behaviour? *Journal of Sport Sciences*, **14**, 18–19.

Bajekal, M. & Purdon, S. (2001) *Social Capital and Social Exclusion: Development of a Condensed Module for the Health Survey of England*. London: National Centre for Social Research.

Bandura, A. (1977) Self-efficacy: toward a unifying theory of behaviour change, *Psychological Review*, **84**, 191–215.

Bandura A. (1986) *Social Foundations of Thought and Action: A Cognitive Social Theory*. Englewood Cliffs, NJ: Prentice Hall.

Bandura, A. (1997) *Self-Efficacy: The Exercise of Control*. New York: Freeman.

Bayly, L. & Bull, F. (2001) *How to Build Social Capital: A Case Study of an Enduring Community Walking Group*. Perth, WA: Eastern Perth Public and Community Health Unit and Department of Public Health, University of Western Australia.

Bekaert, S. (2003) Developing adolescent services in general practice, *Nursing Standard*, **17**, 33–6.

Bergman, A. B., Rivara, F. P., Richards, D. D. & Rogers, L. W. (1990) The Seattle Children's Bicycle Helmet Campaign, *American Journal of Disorders in Children*, **144**, 727–31.

Berkman, L. F. (2000) Social support, social networks, social cohesion and health, *Social Work and Health Care*, **31**, 3–14.

Biddle, S. J. H. & Nigg, C. (2000) Theories of exercise behaviour, *International Journal of Sport Psychology*, **31**, 290–304.

Booth, M. L., Bauman, A., Owen, N. & Gore, C. J. (1997) Physical activity preferences, preferred sources of assistance, and perceived barriers to increased activity among physically inactive Australians, *Preventive Medicine*, **26**, 111–13.

Bourdieu, P. (1977) *Outline of a Theory of Practice*. Cambridge: Cambridge University Press.

Bozionelos, G. & Bennett, P. (1999) The theory of planned behaviour as predictor of exercise, *Journal of Health Psychology*, **4**, 517–29.

Bryman, A. (1988) *Quantity and Quality in Social Research*. Boston: Unwin Hyman.

Bunton, R., Baldwin, S., Flynn, D. & Whitelaw, S. (2000) The 'Stage of Change' model in health promotion: science and ideology, *Critical Public Health*, **10**, 55–70.

Calfas, K. J., Sallis, J. F., Oldenberg, B. & French, M. (1997) Mediators of change in physical activity following an intervention in primary care: PACE, *Preventive Medicine*, **26**, 297–304.

Capibas. (1999) *Attitudes to Fitness. Report JN: 15035*. London: Capibus Omnibus.

Caplan, R. (1993) The importance of social theory for health promotion: from description to reflexivity, *Health Promotion International*, **8**, 147–57.

Cardinal, B. J. & Levy, S. S. (1999) Are sedentary behaviours terminable? *Medicine and Science in Sport and Exercise*, **31** (supplement), S391.

Chapman, G., Adam, S. & Stockford, D. (2001) National Service frameworks; promoting the public health, *Journal of Epidemiology and Community Health*, **55**, 373–4.

Chatzisarantis, N. L. D., Hagger, M. S., Biddle, S. J. H., Karageorghis, C., Smith, B. M. & Sage L. (in press) The influences of perceived autonomy support on physical activity within the theory of planned behaviour, *Journal of Sport and Exercise Psychology*.

Children's Society and Play Council. (2003) Grumpy grown ups stop play, reveals Playday Research. Accessed 27 October, 2003. http://cgi.www. d emon.net/cgi-bin/www.childsoc.org.uk/open.pl?file=/news/news_items/ play_prevention.htm

Chinn, D. J., White, M., Harland, J., Drinkwater, C. & Raybould, S. (1999) Barriers to physical activity and socio-economic position: implications for health promotion, *Journal of Epidemiology and Community Health*, **53**, 191–2.

Cohen, S. & Herbert, T. B. (1996) Psychological factors and physical disease from the perspective of human psychoneuroimmunology, *Annual Review of Psychology*, **47**, 113–42.

Davison, C., Frankl, S. & Davey Smith, G. (1992) The limit of lifestyle: reassessing 'fatalism' in the popular culture of illness prevention, *Social Science and Medicine*, **34**, 675–85.

Diaz, E. M. (2002) Theory of planned behaviour and pedestrians' intentions to violate traffic regulations, *Transportation Research*, **Part F, 5**, 169–75.

Donovan, R. J., Jones, S., D'Arcy, C., Holman, J. & Corti B. (1998) Assessing reliability of a stage of change scale, *Health Education Research*, **13**, 285–91.

Doyal, L. (2003) Gendering health: men, women and well-being. In Sidell, M., Jones, L., Katz, J., Peberdy, A. & Douglas, J. (eds), *Debates and Dilemmas in Promoting Health: A Reader* 2nd edn. Basingstoke: Palgrave Macmillan, 372–82.

Dryden, W. & Feltham, C. (1992) *Brief Counselling: A Practical Guide for Beginning Practitioners*. Buckingham: Open University.

Dunn, A. L., Marcus, B. H., Kampert, J. B., Garcia, M. E., Kohl, H. W., & Blair, S. N. (1997) Reduction in cardiovascular disease risk factors: 6-month results from Project Active, *Preventive Medicine*, **26**, 883–92.

Emmons, K. M. & Rollnick, S. (2001) Motivational interviewing in health care settings; opportunities and limitations, *American Journal of Preventive Medicine*, **20**, 68–74.

Engel, R. J., Rose, J. S., Yanessa, J. F., Raglin, J. & Mannix, E. T. (1999) Applying the transtheoretical model to predict exercise level among physically active adults, *Medicine and Science in Sports and Exercise*, **31**(supplement), S391.

Eves, F., Mant, S. & Clarke, P. (1996) Barriers to exercise at different stages of exercise behaviour, *Journal of Sports Sciences*, **14**, 29.

Fahrenwald, N. L. & Walker, S. N. (2003) Application of the transtheoretical model of behaviour change to the physical activity behaviour of WIC mothers, *Public Health Nursing*, **20**, 307–17.

Finch, C. F., McIntosh, A. S. & McCrory, P. (2001) What do under 15 year-old schoolboy rugby union players think about protective headgear? *British Journal of Sports Medicine*, **35**, 89–94.

Fishbein, M. & Ajzen, I. (1975) *Belief, Attitude, Intention, and Behavior: An Introduction to Theory and Research.* Reading, MA: Addison-Wesley.

Fitness Industry Association. (2000) *Why People Quit.* London: Fitness Industry Association.

Freudenberg, N., Eng, E., Flay, B., Parcel, G., Rogers, T. & Wallerstein, N. (1995) Strengthening individual and community capacity to prevent disease and promote health: in search of relevant theories and principles, *Health Education Quarterly*, **22**, 290–306.

Garfield, S. L. (1994) Research on client variables in psychotherapy. In Garfield, S. L. & Bergin, A. E. (eds), *Handbook of Psychotherapy and Behavior Change*, 4th edn. New York: Wiley & Sons.

Giddens, A. (1984) *The Constitution of Society.* Cambridge: Polity Press.

Gorely, T. & Bruce, D. (2000) A 6-month investigation of exercise adoption from the contemplation stage of the transtheoretical model, *Psychology of Sport and Exercise*, **1**, 89–101.

Gunaratnam, Y. (2003) More than word: dialogue across difference. In Sidell, M., Jones, L., Katz, J., Peberdy, A. & Douglas, J. (eds), *Debates and Dilemmas in Promoting Health: A Reader*, 2nd edn. Basingstoke: Palgrave Macmillan, 112–21.

Heesch, K. C., Brown, D. R. & Blanton, C. J. (1999) Perceived barriers to exercise and stage of exercise adoption in older minority and Caucasian women, *Medicine and Science in Sport and Exercise*, **31**(supplement), S185.

Hewstone, M. (1989) *Causal Attribution: From Cognitive Processes to Collective Beliefs.* Oxford: Blackwell.

Hillman, M., Adams, J. & Whitelegg, J. (1991) *One False Move . . . A Study of Children's Independent Mobility.* London: Policy Studies Institute.

Hillsdon, M., Cavill, N. K., Nanchahal, K., Diamond, A. & White, I. R. (2001) National level promotion of physical activity: results from England's Active for Life campaign, *Journal of Epidemiology and Community Health*, **55**, 755–61.

Jaffee, L., Lutter, J. M., Rex, J., Hawkes, C. & Bucaccio, P. (1999) Incentives and barriers to physical activity for working women, *American Journal of Health Promotion*, **13**, 215–18.

Janis, I. L. & Mann, L. (1977) *Decision Making.* New York: Free Press.

Jordan, P. J., Nigg, C. R., Norman, G. J., Rossi, J. S. & Benisovich, S. V. (2002) Does the transtheoretical model need an attitude adjustment? Integrating attitude with decisional balance as predictors of stage of change for exercise, *Psychology of Sport and Exercise*, **3**, 65–83.

Kennedy, M. F. & Meeuwisse, W. H. (2003) Exercise counselling by family physicians in Canada, *Preventive Medicine*, **37**, 226–32.

Kerlinger, F. (1986) *The Foundations of Behavioural Research*. New York: Holt, Rinehart & Winston.

Kerr, J. & McKenna, J. (2000) A randomised control trial of advertising to promote walking, *Journal of Health Communication*, **5**, 265–79.

Kiecolt-Glaser, J. K., Kennedy, S., Malkoff, S., Fisher, L., Speicher, C. E., & Glaser, R. (1988) Marital discord and immunity in males, *Psychosomatic Medicine*, **50**, 213–29.

Kiecolt-Glaser, J. K., McGuire, L., Robles, T. F. & Glaser, R. (2002) Emotions, morbidity and mortality: new perspectives from psychoneuroimmunology, *Annual Review of Psychology*, **53**, 83–107.

Klar, Y., Nadler, A., & Malloy, T. E. (1992) Opting to change; students' informal self-change endeavours. In Klar, Y., Nadler, A. & Malloy, T. E. (eds), *Self Change: Social Psychological and Clinical Perspectives*. New York: Springer-Verlag, 63–83.

Krantz, D. S. & McCeney, M. K. (2002) Effects of psychological and social factors on organic disease: a critical assessment of research on coronary heart disease, *Annual Review of Psychology*, **53**, 341–69.

Kreuter, M. W., Lukwago, S. N., Bucholtz, D. C., Clark, E. M. & Sanders-Thompson, V. (2003) Achieving cultural appropriateness in health promotion programs: targeted and tailored approaches, *Health Education and Behaviour*, **30**, 133–46.

Kuh, D. & Ben-Shlomo, Y. (eds) (1997) *A Lifecourse Approach to Chronic Disease Epidemiology*. Oxford: Oxford University Press.

Kumanyika, S. K. (2003) Commentary: cultural appropriateness: working our way toward a practicable framework, *Health Education and Behaviour*, **30**, 147–50.

Larimer, M. E. & Marlatt, G. A. (1992) Determinants of relapse in addictive behaviours: a social learning approach to facilitating maintenance. In Klar, Y., Fisher, J. D., Chinsky, J. M. & Nadler, A. (eds), *Self Change: Social Psychological and Clinical Perspectives*. New York: Springer-Verlag, 137–51.

Lee, R. E. & Cubbin, C. (2002) Neighborhood context and youth cardiovascular health behaviours, *American Journal of Public Health*, **92**, 428–36.

Leslie, E., Johnson-Kozlow, M., Sallis, J. F., Owen, N. & Bauman, A. (2003) Reliability of moderate-intensity and vigorous physical activity stage of change measures for young adults, *Preventive Medicine*, **37**, 177–81.

Macdonald, M. A. & Green, L. W. (2001) Reconciling concept and context: the dilemma of implementation in school-based health promotion, *Health Education and Behaviour*, **28**, 749–68.

Marcus, B. H., Dunn, A. L., Kampert, J. B., Barlow, C. E. & Blair, S. N. (2000) Project PRIME: six-month changes in behavioural processes predict increases in physical activity, *Medicine and Science in Sports and Exercise*, **32**(supplement), S253.

Marcus, B. H., Rakowski, W. & Rossi, J. (1992) Assessing motivational readiness and decision making for exercise, *Health Psychology*, **11**, 257–61.

Marcus, B. H., Selby, V., Niaura, R. & Rossi, J. S. (1992) Self-efficacy and the stages of exercise behaviour change, *Research Quarterly for Exercise and Sport*, **63**, 60–6.

Marcus, B. H. & Stanton, A. L. (1993) Evaluation of relapse prevention and reinforcement interventions to promote exercise adherence in sedentary females, *Research Quarterly for Exercise and Sport*, **64**, 447–52.

Marmot, M., Bosma, H., Hemingway, E. et al. (1997) Contribution of job control and other risk factors to social variations in coronary heart disease incidence, *The Lancet*, **350**, 235–39.

McEwan, B. & Stellar, E. (1993) Stress and the individual. Mechanisms leading to disease, *Archives of Internal Medicine*, **1563**, 2093–103.

McKenna, J. & Francis, C. (2003) Exercise contemplators: unravelling the processes of change, *Health Education*, **103**, 41–53.

McKenna, J. & Vernon, M. (in press) How general practitioners promote 'lifestyle' physical activity, *Patient Education and Counseling*.

McKenna, J. & Whatley, M. (in press) 'If only they'd treat me like a man on a horse': experiences of commuter cycling, *Journal of Sport Sciences*.

Merzel, C. & D'Afflitti, J. (2003) Reconsidering community-based health promotion: promise, performance and potential, *American Journal of Public Health*, **93**, 557–74.

Miller, W. R. & Rollnick, S. (1991) In Miller W. R. & Rollnick, S. (eds), *Motivational Interviewing: Preparing People to Change Addictive Behaviour*. New York: Guilford Press.

Naylor, P. J. & McKenna, J. (1995) Stages of change, self-efficacy and behavioural preferences for exercise among British university students, *Journal of Sports Science*, **13**, 68.

Nigg, C. & Courneya, K. (1998) Transtheoretical model: examining adolescent exercise behavior, *Journal of Adolescent Health*, **22**, 214–24.

O'Connell, B. (1998) *Solution-Focused Therapy*. London: Sage.

Pinto, B. M., Goldstein, M. G. & Marcus, B. H. (1998) Activity counseling by primary care physicians, *Preventive Medicine*, **27**, 506–13.

Plotnikoff, R. C., Hotz, S. B., Birkett, N. J. & Courneya, K. S. (2001) Exercise and the transtheoretical model: a longitudinal test of a population sample, *Preventive Medicine*, **33**, 441–52.

Plotnikoff, R. C., Hotz, S. B., Birkett, N. J., Hanson, J. S. & Leonard, L. E. (1999) Explaining energy expenditure and stages of change: a longitudinal population study, *Medicine and Science in Sport and Exercise*, **31**(supplement), S186.

Prochaska, J. O. (1994) Strong and weak principles for progressing from pre-contemplation to action on the basis of twelve problem behaviours, *Health Psychology*, **13**, 47–51.

Prochaska, J. O. (1999) Prescribing to the stages and levels of change, *Psychotherapy*, **28**, 463–68.

Prochaska, J. O. & DiClemente, C. C. (1982) Transtheoretical therapy: toward a more integrative model of change, *Psychotherapy, Therapy, Research and Practice*, **19**, 276–88.

Prochaska, J. O. & DiClemente, C. C. (1992) In search of how people change: applications to addictive behaviours, *American Psychologist*, **47**, 1102–14.

Prochaska, J. O. & DiClemente, C. C. (1994) *The Transtheoretical Approach: Crossing Traditional Boundaries of Therapy*. Malabar, FA: Krieger.

Prochaska, J., Norcross, J. C. & DiClemente, C. C. (1996) *Changing for Good*. New York: Avon.

Putnam, R. D. (2000) *Bowling Alone*. New York: Simon and Schuster.

Quine, L. Rutter, D. R. & Arnold, L. (2001) Persuading school-aged cyclists to use safety helmets: effectiveness of an intervention based on the theory of planned behaviour, *British Journal of Health Psychology*, **6**, 327–45.

Raphael, D. (2000) The question of evidence in health promotion, *Health Promotion International*, **15**, 355–67.

Ratner, H. & Yandoli, D. (1996) Solution focused brief therapy: a co-operative approach to work with clients. In Edwards, G. & Dare, C. (eds), *Psychotherapy, Psychological Treatments and the Addictions*. Cambridge: Cambridge University Press, 124–38.

Reed, G. R. (1999) Adherence to exercise and the transtheoretical model of behaviour change. In Bull, S. J. (ed.), *Adherence Issues in Sport and Exercise*. Chichester: John Wiley and Sons, 19–45.

Repetti, R. L., McGrath, E. P. & Ishikawa, S. S. (1996) Daily stress and coping in childhood and adolescence. In Goreczny, A. J., & Hersen, M. (eds), *Handbook of Pediatric and Adolescent Health Psychology*. Boston: Allyn & Bacon.

Riddoch, C. J. (1998) Relationships between physical activity and physical health in young people. In Biddle, S., Sallis, J. & Cavill, N. (eds), *Young and Active? Young People and Health-Enhancing Physical Activity – Evidence and Implications*. London: Health Education Authority, 17–48.

Rollnick, S. & Miller, W. (1995) What is motivational interviewing? *Behavioural and Cognitive Psychotherapy*, **23**, 325–34.

Rosal, M. C., Ebbeling, C. B., Lofgren, I., Ockene, J. K., Ockene, O. S. & Herbert, J. R. (2001) Facilitating dietary change: The patient-centred counseling approach. Journal of the American Dietetic Association, **101**, 332–8, 341.

Rosen, C. S. (2000) Integrating stage and continuum models to explain processing of exercise messages and exercise initiation among sedentary college students, *Health Psychology*, **19**, 172–80.

Rothman, A. J. (2000) Toward a theory-based analysis of behavioural maintenance, *Health Psychology*, **19**(supplement), 64–9.

Sallis, J. F. & Owen N. (1999) *Physical Activity & Behavioral Medicine*. Berkeley, CA: Sage.

Sarkin, J. A., Johnson, S. S., Prochaska, J. O. & Prochaska, J. M. (2001) Applying the transtheoretical model to regular moderate exercise in an overweight population: validation of a stages of change measure, *Preventive Medicine*, **33**, L462–9.

Schneider Jamner, M. (2000) Introduction. In Schneider Jamner, M. & Stokols, D. (eds), *Promoting Human Wellness*. Berkeley, CA: University of California Press, ch. 1.

Scogin, F., Bynum, J., Stephens, G. & Calhoon, S. (1990) Efficacy of self-administered treatment programs: meta-analytic review, *Professional Psychology: Research and Practice*, **21**, 42–7.

Seedhouse, D. (1997) *Health Promotion: Philosophy, Prejudice and Practice*. New York: John Wiley.

Shinn, M. & Toohey, S. M. (2003) Community context of human welfare, *Annual Review of Psychology*, **54**, 427–59.

Siegler, J. C., Peterson, B. L., Barefoot, J. C. & Williams, R. B. (1992) Hostility during late adolescence predicts coronary risk factors at mid-life, *American Journal of Epidemiology*, **136**, 146–54.

Silver-Wallace L., Buckworth, J., Kirby, T. E. & Sherman, W. M. (2000) Characteristics of exercise behavior among college students: application of social cognitive theory to predicting stage of change, *Preventive Medicine*, **31**, 494–505.

Spence, J. C. & Lee, R. E. (2003) Toward a comprehensive model of physical activity, *Psychology of Sport and Exercise*, **4**, 7–24.

Sports Council & Health Education Authority (1992) *Allied Dunbar National Fitness Survey*. London: Sports Council & Health Education Authority.

Steptoe, A., Wardle, J., Fuller, R., Holte, A., Justo, J., Sanderman, R. & Wichstrøm, L. (1997) Leisure-time physical exercise: prevalence, attitudinal correlates, and behavioral correlates among young Europeans from 21 countries, *Preventive Medicine*, **26**, 845–54.

Syme, L. S. (2000) Community participation, empowerment and health. In Schneider Jamner, M. & Stokols, D. (eds), *Promoting Human Wellness*. Berkeley, CA: University of California Press, 78–98.

Theodorakis, Y. (1994) Planned behaviour; attitude strength, role identify, and the prediction of exercise behaviour, *The Sport Psychologist*, **8**, 149–65.

Velicer, W. F., DiClemente, C. C., Rossi, J. S. & Prochaska, J. O. (1990) Relapse situations and self-efficacy: an integrative model, *Addictive Behaviours*, **15**, 271–83.

Walker, Z., Townsend, J., Oakley, L., Donovan, C., Smith, H., Hurst, Z. et al. (2002) Health promotion for adolescents in primary care: randomised controlled trial, *British Medical Journal*, **325**, 524–30.

Walker, Z. A. K. & Townsend, J. (1999) The role of general practice in promoting teenage health: a review of the literature, *Family Practice*, **16**, 164–72.

Wankel, L. & Mummery, W. (1993) Using national survey data incorporating the theory of planned behaviour: implications for social marketing strategies in physical activity, *Journal of Applied Sport Psychology*, **5**, 158–77.

Weinstein, N. D., Rothman, A. J. & Sutton, S. R. (1998) Stage theories of health behaviour: conceptual and methodological issues, *Health Psychology*, **17**, 290–9.

Whitehead, M. (1997) How useful is the 'stages of change' model? *Health Education Journal*, **56**, 111–12.

Wing, R. R. (2000) Cross-cutting themes in maintenance of behaviour change, *Health Psychology*, **19**(supplement), 84–8.

Witte, K. & Allen, M. (2000) A meta-analysis of fear appeals: implications for effective public health campaigns, *Health Education and Behaviour*, **27**, 591–615.

Zhu, W. & Ainsworth, B. E. (1999) Validation of a classification algorithm of stage of change in an urban women population, *Medicine and Science in Sport and Exercise*, **31**(supplement), S95.

7

Promoting Physical Activity within Schools

Lorraine Cale and Jo Harris

Given the concerns over the physical activity levels of many young people, targeted efforts to promote physical activity are clearly vital. In this respect, the role of the school in the promotion of physical activity has attracted increased interest in recent years and schools have been acknowledged as the primary institution with responsibility for promoting activity in young people (McBride & Midford, 1999; Sallis & Owen, 1999; Cardon & De Bourdeaudhuij, 2002). More specifically, school physical education (PE) has been recognized as having a key role to play (see, for example, Cale, 2000a; Shephard & Trudeau, 2000; McKenzie, 2001; Armstrong, 2000; Cardon & De Bourdeaudhuij, 2002). Green (2002, p. 95) refers to the 'taken-for-granted role of PE in health promotion', and McKenzie (2001) views PE as the most suitable vehicle for the promotion of active, healthy lifestyles among young people.

Furthermore, the role of schools and PE in promoting health and the link between health and education has increasingly been recognized by government. Green (2002) reports that encouraging participation in sport and physical activity has been a persistent and enduring theme of government policy towards school sport and PE in recent decades and how a range of publications have attested to the desirability of utilizing PE in order to promote lifelong participation in (sport) and physical activity (e.g. DoH, 1999; DCMS, 2001). Similarly, Harris & Penney (2000, p. 252) note how official and semi-official pronouncements on behalf of government have clearly identified PE as 'critical in educating and providing opportunities for young people to become independently active for life'. Perhaps the most recent and significant example of this has been the launch of the PE, School Sport and Club Links Strategy. The strategy, which is outlined in more detail in Chapter 10, was launched in October 2002 and is being delivered by the DfES (Department for Education and Skills) and DCMS (Department for Culture, Media and Sport) and supported by a government investment of £459 million over three years (DfES, 2003).

This chapter, then, explores the role and potential that schools and PE have for promoting physical activity both within and beyond the curriculum, and considers some of the major issues and considerations relating to the promotion of physical activity within this context. Whilst much of the discussion focuses on the curriculum and developments in schools in the UK, the issues raised are considered equally relevant and applicable to most other developed countries.

Discussion point   To what extent do you feel that schools should be concerned with physical activity promotion?

Who should be responsible for and involved in physical activity promotion in schools?

What opportunities are there for physical activity promotion in schools?

What constraints are there to physical activity promotion in schools?

The school is considered an appropriate setting for the promotion of health-related behaviours, including physical activity, for a number of reasons. Fox & Harris suggest that schools:

- offer one of the few settings where the full socio-economic spectrum is both represented and in attendance, and where sustained exposure to healthy messages and health expertise can be achieved;
- occupy a good deal of the time of youngsters – the school can influence the behaviour of children for about 40–45 per cent of their waking time;
- have a primary function to provide a context for learning at a time of development that is characterized by high receptiveness. (2003, p. 182)

In addition, over the years and more recently under the 1996 Education Act, schools are required to provide a balanced and broadly-based curriculum which promotes the spiritual, cultural, mental and *physical* development of pupils. Schools can also have a wider impact beyond young people and can influence teachers, ancillary staff, governors and parents (Cale, 1997). Finally, and as Chapter 10 reveals, school-based intervention studies can achieve positive results and influence young people's health, fitness and physical activity levels, as well as knowledge, understanding and attitudes towards physical activity (Harris & Cale 1997; Almond & Harris, 1998; Cale & Harris, 1998; Stone et al., 1998).

Developments in health-enhancing physical activity

Maintaining health through PE is not a new concept. Indeed, PE was driven by this objective at the beginning of the twentieth century (Sleap, 1990). However, by the end of the Second World War other objectives of PE came to the fore, at the expense of a concern for health. Attention shifted more towards self-discovery and the acquisition of physical skills, and it was not until the early 1980s that health once again became an important objective of the PE curriculum. Since this time, the emphasis and interest has continued to flourish, and there has been a documented and active interest by many PE teachers in promoting health-related physical activity in schools in the UK (Williams, 1988). During the latter part of the 80s, Almond (1989) pointed to a virtual tenfold rise in the number of schools incorporating a health-based approach within their PE programme.

The movement was then given some consideration in the drafting of the first NCPE (National Curriculum for Physical Education) in 1992 and HRE (health-related exercise), as the area commonly became termed, was included as a statutory component of the NCPE (DES & WO, 1992) and a component of the cross-curricular theme of health education (NCC, 1990). For the first time, it was formally recognized and had a specific knowledge base and place in the curriculum. However, while the NCPE brought with it a formal requirement that health issues should be addressed, its position and mode of expression in the curriculum were vague (Harris, 1997a). To the disappointment of many, the area was not afforded the status of a separate programme of study but it was identified as a theme to be delivered through the activity areas. This received some criticism and it was feared that without a formal programme, the area could easily be marginalized or overlooked (Fox, 1992; Cale, 1996; Penney & Evans, 1997). Furthermore, following a national survey of HRE in 1000 secondary schools, Harris (1997a) revealed the teaching of health-related activity in PE to be characterized by confusion, limited systematic expression, considerable variation in practice, and inconsistent and insufficient guidance for teachers. In short, health promotion as a key goal of physical education remained neither universally accepted nor well understood (Harris, 1995).

More recently, and on a more positive note, subsequent revisions of the NCPE (DfE and WO, 1995; DfEE & QCA, 1999a) have provided a stronger positioning of health-related issues which implies a more explicit prompt for the area to be addressed in curriculum planning and delivery (Fox & Harris, 2003).

In the meantime, and in response to concerns over the value, content, expression, delivery and organization of health-based work within the curriculum, and teachers' relatively limited knowledge and understanding of the area (Fox, 1992; Cale, 1996; Almond & Harris, 1997; Harris, 1997a), a Health-Related Exercise Working Group, comprising representatives from schools, higher education, the advisory service and key sport, health and PE organizations, was established in 1997 in an effort to establish a consensus approach to the area. The main task of the group was to produce good practice guidelines for teachers in the form of a curriculum resource. Following consultation, the Guidance Material was published in 2000 (Harris, 2000) to coincide with, and support teachers in the delivery of the revised NCPE.

A further development of significance was the launch of the HEA's (now the HDA (Health Development Agency)) policy framework for the promotion of health-enhancing physical activity for young people, *Young and Active?*, in June 1998 (HEA, 1998) (see Chapter 5). The framework identifies the education sector as one of the key organizations which has a role to play in promoting health-enhancing physical activity, and includes a series of recommendations as to how schools can promote physical activity to young people.

Finally, and as was highlighted earlier, encouraging participation in sport and physical activity has been a focus of government policy in recent years and there has been a call from government for the broadening of provision within the PE curriculum to enhance lifelong learning and healthy lifestyles. In the first instance, this led to the removal of the compulsory requirement to study games activities for 14–16-year-olds (DfEE & QCA, 1999a). More recently, with the launch of the PE, School Sport and Club Links Strategy, measures are now being taken to increase the percentage of young people in England who spend a minimum of two hours in PE and school sport per week. In order to achieve this, a range of further initiatives and programmes are being implemented, the details of which are outlined in Chapter 10. All of the above are encouraging developments that have the potential to enhance the future provision and quality of health-enhancing physical activity in schools.

Promoting physical activity within the curriculum

There is no doubt that the PE curriculum has a key role to play in providing appropriate physical activity opportunities, information and guidance to young people, and in encouraging and empowering young people to make informed lifestyle choices. How specifically, though, the PE curriculum can promote physical activity warrants consideration.

The National Curriculum

'The government believes that two hours of physical activity a week, including the National Curriculum for Physical Education and extra-curricular activities, should be an aspiration for all schools' (DfEE & QCA, 1999b, p. 17).

The National Curriculum for England comprises statutory programmes of study for PE (covering athletic activities, dance activities, games activities, gymnastic activities, outdoor and adventurous activities, and swimming activities and water safety), four aspects in PE in which pupils make progress, including knowledge and understanding of *fitness and health*, and a non-statutory framework for PSHE (personal, social and health education) (DfEE & QCA, 1999a; 1999b). The National Curriculum for Wales is similar in that it comprises programmes of study for PE and a framework for PSE (personal and social, education) (ACCAC, 2000a; 2000b). Further, the NCPE for Wales states that HRE should be taught at each Key Stage and one of the four areas of experience within the Key Stage 4 programme of study is exercise activities (i.e. non-competitive forms of exercise such as step aerobics, jogging, weight training, cycling, circuit training and skipping).

More recently, the Guidance Material produced by Harris (2000) has provided an interpretation of these requirements for teachers. The interpretation is expressed in the form of learning outcomes for each Key Stage that address the health and fitness requirements of the PE curriculum and incorporate links with relevant health-related aspects of PSHE and Science (Harris, 2000). The learning outcomes have been placed into four categories, namely (1) safety issues, (2) exercise effects, (3) health benefits and (4) activity promotion to clarify the range of coverage and the progression between Key Stages.

HRE interpretation, organization and delivery

As highlighted earlier, concerns have been expressed over the inconsistent and limited approach to HRE in the past, and interpretations, organization and delivery of the area have varied (Harris, 2000; Fox & Harris, 2003). According to Harris (1997b), HRE means different things to different people and it is therefore important to clarify exactly what is meant by the term. The most commonly accepted definition states that, within the context of the NCPE, HRE relates to 'the teaching of knowledge, understanding, physical competence and behavioural skills, and the creation of positive attitudes and confidence associated with current and lifelong participation in physical activity' (Harris, 2000, p. 2).

HRE is physical activity associated with health enhancement and should involve learning through active participation in purposeful activity embracing a range of sport, dance and exercise experiences including individualized lifetime activities.

Research, however, has highlighted examples of narrow interpretations of HRE that often equate the area with some or all of the following: vigorous activity such as cross-country running (in which young people are forced to 'huff and puff' or 'heave and pull'); fitness testing; safety and hygiene issues such as warming up and cooling down, lifting and carrying equipment, and showers (Harris, 1997b). Such narrow interpretations are a concern in that they have the potential to lead to undesirable practices such as forced fitness regimes, directed activity with minimal learning, inactive PE lessons involving excessive theory or teacher talk, or dull, uninspiring drills (Harris, 2000). Furthermore, some teachers fail to recognize the knowledge base associated with HRE and merely deliver activity-based units (e.g. blocks of aerobics, cross-country) without imparting learning. Evidence also suggests that physiological issues, such as the physical effects of exercise and fitness testing, have dominated HRE courses in schools (Harris, 1995; 2000).

Equally, the belief that HRE is purely a matter of transmitting information and knowledge to young people and telling them to be more active is a mistaken one. It is commonly accepted within health promotion that knowledge alone is insufficient to bring about behaviour change (Douthitt & Harvey, 1995) and that simply encouraging children to be more active takes no account of the socio-cultural, environmental and behavioural factors influencing children's participation in activity (Smith & Biddle, 1995). Yet, according to Smith & Biddle (1995) and Harris (1995; 2000), limited attention is paid to such factors in the school curriculum.

The National Curriculum specifies content, not delivery, and it therefore allows scope for professional judgment regarding how best to transmit content, including knowledge and understanding of fitness and health, within the context of different schools (Harris & Almond, 1994; Harris 1997b). The responsibility of schools and teachers is to deliver the statutory requirements of the NCPE effectively and Harris (1997b) reminds us that the critical issue is the effectiveness of the learning more than the particular approach adopted. Nonetheless, there has been considerable debate in recent years concerning the way in which HRE should be organized within the curriculum (Fox, 1992; Harris & Elbourn, 1992; Almond & Harris, 1997; Harris, 1997b; Stratton, 1998). Various approaches are possible, including permeation or integrated, focused, topic, and combined, and each has specific strengths and limitations (see Table 7.1). The absence of an activity area for HRE in the NCPE has been interpreted by some to indicate that HRE should be delivered solely through the activity areas (via permeation), rather than in discrete blocks or units of work (Oxley, 1994). As Table 7.1 implies, however, this model can be rather 'hit and miss'. Furthermore, such an approach may deny young people the opportunity to engage in a variety of popular health-promoting lifetime exercise activities (Fox & Harris, 2003).

Research conducted by Harris (1995) and Cale (2000a) has revealed the most common approach to be through a combination of approaches (i.e. focused units of work in PE, integration through the activity areas, and delivery within other areas of the curriculum) which suggests that value is being placed on HRE in many schools and that a number of teachers are taking the time to plan, structure, implement and co-ordinate the area. Curriculum leaders and heads of PE who are familiar with their own curriculum, colleagues and pupils are clearly in the best position to make appropriate decisions concerning which approach or approaches to adopt, based on the strengths and limitations of each approach.

In terms of the delivery of HRE, the following desirable and undesirable practices have been identified (Harris, 2000, p. 17):

HRE	Desirable practices	Undesirable practices
Status	Explicit, valued, planned, evaluated	Implicit, low status, incidental, not monitored
Breadth and relevance	Comprehensive, meaningful, focus on health/activity/ participation	Narrow, superficial, emphasis on fitness testing/hard training/elite performance

Coherence and status	Coherent, co-ordinated, clear links with PE activity areas/PSHE and related subjects, integrated	Ad hoc, hit and miss, limited links with PE activity areas/PSHE and related subjects
Equity	Inclusive, involving all pupils	Exclusive, reduced or minimal involvement of pupils such as the least active, less competent and those with disabilities and health conditions
Action	Requires guidance and support	Requires change

Research suggests, however, that many schools may be falling short of achieving the desirable practices. For example, studies by Harris (1995) and Cale (2000a) revealed that only approximately a third and a half of schools, respectively, considered the teaching of HRE in their schools to be fully structured. Harris (1997a) also noted that the way that many health-related programmes are designed, taught and evaluated in schools continues to be oriented more towards 'fitness for sports performance' than 'fitness for healthy lifestyles', whereas Harris and Penney (2000) found that, rather than promoting equity and inclusion, health-related PE programmes often reflect, express and reinforce gendered practices through 'female' and 'male' versions of HRE.

Furthermore, the way in which HRE information and activity experiences are presented is critical. Regardless of the approach adopted, in order to encourage young people to develop a pattern of regular activity, it is important that HRE involves enjoyable, positive and meaningful exercise experiences, a practical knowledge base and caring teaching strategies (Fox & Harris, 2003).

In addition, in promoting physical activity within the curriculum there needs to be an emphasis on the beneficial short- and long-term effects of exercise, improved functional capacity, weight management and psychological wellbeing associated with exercise participation. Highlighting the risks of inactivity (hypokinetic diseases) and threats of illness and death will do little to promote physical activity with young people. As Fox (1993) notes, teenagers believe that they are either immortal or immune from such problems. It is also important that young people be helped to shift from dependence on the teacher to

Table 7.1 Approaches to HRE within the curriculum

Approach	Strengths	Limitations
Permeation An approach in which HRE is taught through the PE activity areas (i.e. through athletics, dance, games, gymnastics, outdoor and adventurous activities, and swimming).	HRE knowledge, understanding and skills can be seen as part of and integral to all PE experiences. Children learn that all physical activities can contribute towards good health and can become part of an active lifestyle.	HRE knowledge, understanding and skills may become lost or marginalised amongst other information relating to skills and performance. Pupils may be overloaded with information. Much liaison activity is required to ensure that all pupils receive similar information from different teachers. The approach may be somewhat ad hoc and piecemeal.
Focused/Discrete An approach involving teaching HRE through specific focused lessons or units of work within either a PE or PSE–PSHE programme.	A specific focus can help ensure that HRE does not become lost or take second place to other information. HRE is less likely to be regarded as an assumed by-product of PE lessons, and HRE is perceived as important through having its own time slot and identity. The value and status of the associated knowledge, understanding and skills are raised.	HRE may be seen in isolation and not closely linked to the PE activity areas. The HRE knowledge, understanding and skills may be delivered over a period of time with long gaps in between, which is problematic in terms of cohesion and progression (e.g. one short block of work per year). The knowledge base may be delivered in such a way as to reduce activity levels within PE lessons (e.g. too much teacher talk).

Topic
An approach involving a series of lessons following a specific topic or theme that is taught through PE and classroom lessons. This may incorporate both permeation and focused units.

HRE may be delivered in a more holistic manner with closer links to other health behaviours (such as eating a balanced diet) and other national curriculum subjects. The area can be covered in more depth and be closely related to pupils' personal experiences. The amount of time engaged in physical activity in PE lessons might be increased if introductory and follow-up work is conducted in the classroom.

A topic or theme-based approach may be more time-consuming with respect to planning. This approach could be less practically oriented than other approaches (if it incorporates a high degree of classroom based work).

Combined
Any combination of permeation, focused and topic-based approaches is possible.

This builds on the strengths of each approach. It ensures that value is placed on HRE and that the area of work is closely linked to all PE experiences and other health behaviours and related subjects.

Combined approaches initially may be more time-consuming to plan, structure, implement and co-ordinate within the curriculum.

Source: Health-related Exercise in the National Curriculum Key Stages 1 to 4. Copyright © 2000 by Jo Harris. By permission of Human Kinetics, Champaign, IL, USA.

independence, by acquiring the necessary understanding, competence and confidence to be active independently (Harris, 2000).

Promoting physical activity within the whole school

The need to move beyond the curriculum and to promote physical activity through other avenues of the school has been increasingly recognized in recent years (Biddle, 1991; Fox, 1996; Cale, 1997; 2000a; 2000b; Cardon & De Bourdeaudhuij, 2002; Fox & Harris, 2003). Fox & Harris (2003), for example, claim that the focus on PE provides only one part of the solution – it represents much less than 2 per cent of the child's waking time and therefore can not in itself address activity shortfalls. Similarly, Cale (1997; 2000a) claims that the curriculum is a vitally important avenue for promoting physical activity, but that this is just one of many aspects of the school that impact upon young people.

Within the curriculum, teachers typically adopt educational or behavioural approaches to the promotion of physical activity, presenting persuasive arguments for and relevant information about physical activity, and possibly involving pupils in learning self-management and regulatory skills such as goal setting, programme planning, self-reinforcement and monitoring or time management to encourage participation in physical activity. Indeed, these skills are considered critical to lifestyle change and activity independence (Corbin, 2002). However, they target only the individual, tend to hold the individual responsible for his or her activity behaviour, and fail to acknowledge other factors in the social environment which influence physical activity (see Chapter 4). Teachers may make young people aware of environmental influences on their behaviour through the curriculum (though as previously highlighted, evidence suggests that few do so), but the curriculum is virtually powerless in terms of being able to address these wider issues. In recognition of such limitations, there has been growing interest and support for environmental or ecological approaches to physical activity promotion in recent years (Sallis, Bauman & Pratt, 1998) (see Chapters 4 and 6). From an environmental perspective, many aspects of the school can either promote or inhibit the adoption of an active lifestyle and understanding gained through the 'formal' curriculum can either be reinforced and supported or completely undermined by the 'hidden curriculum'. A school with poorly maintained playgrounds or playing fields and 'no ball game' policies at breaktimes and lunchtimes, for example, would suggest that it does not value physical activity for pupils. Thus, to increase the likelihood of physical activity promotion being successful and leading to sustainable behaviour change, it should be seen as more than just a curriculum activity focusing on individual behaviour change strategies (Cale, 1997). Instead, the potential of every aspect of the school to promote physical activity should be explored. Examples of relevant whole-school approaches include the Healthy or Health-Promoting School and the Active School.

The Healthy School

The idea of focusing on the school as a health-promoting environment first became popular in the 1980s (Tones & Tilford, 1994) and is now well established. Principally, a Health-Promoting or Healthy School aims to achieve healthy lifestyles for the entire school population (pupils, staff, governors, parents) by developing supportive environments conducive to the promotion of health. Traditionally, three consistent elements have formed the basis of a Health-Promoting School: the curriculum, environment (hidden curriculum) and the wider community (outreach) (Nutbeam, 1992) and a Healthy School would be expected to make explicit its commitment to health by highlighting through its curricular, extra-curricular and organizational practices those aspects of learning which promote good health (Cale, 1997; Harris, 2000).

Government policy in the UK has consistently supported the notion of a Health-Promoting or Healthy School (DoH, 1992; DfEE, 1997; DoH, 1999) resulting in May 1998 in the launch of the Healthy Schools Programme. The programme is a key part of the Government's drive to improve standards of health and education and to tackle health inequalities. It aims to raise awareness of the opportunities in schools for improving health, both physical and mental, of children, teachers, as well as for families and the local community, and encourages schools to develop a 'healthy school' ethos and to develop and improve school and community links.

The Healthy Schools Programme has a national network – the Wired for Health website: www.wiredforhealth.gov.uk Other components of the programme include the National Healthy School Standard and a National Healthy Schools Newsletter. See Chapter 10 for further details about the programme.

The Active School

Although it is now possible to achieve formal recognition as an 'Active School', still comparatively limited attention appears to have been paid to the concept. According to Fox (1996), an Active School is aware of the need to promote physical activity in all children and will constantly be developing strategies that will provide children with activity opportunities and increase their desire and knowledge base to sustain active lifestyles. In short, an Active School will maximize opportunities for children (and all who are associated with the school) to be active by exploring all opportunities and avenues to promote physical activity (Cale, 1997). Therefore, just as a Health-Promoting School is expected to make explicit its commitment to health by high-lighting through its curricular, extra-curricular and organizational practices those aspects of learning which promote good health, an Active School should make a commitment to physical activity and promote active living through the same channels. Likewise, the same elements of the curriculum, environment and the wider community are important in an Active School.

However, there is no single formula for the operation of a successful Active School and there are many ways to become an Active School. Despite this, the formulation of policy or 'policy-making machinery' to ensure that activity promotion remains on the school agenda, and an 'Active School Committee' to develop strategies and goals for increas-ing physical activity and to drive, co-ordinate and evaluate physical activity initiatives are recommended as a sound starting point (Cale, 1997; Harris, 2000; Fox & Harris, 2003).

A number of 'Active School' ideas and strategies have been proposed (for example, see Fox, 1996; Cale, 1997; Fox & Harris, 2003; the Young@ Heart campaign documents (National Heart Forum, 2002)). Cale (1997) presented such strategies in the form of an Active School model which identified seven major avenues through which physical activity could be promoted in schools. A revised version of the model which incorporates ideas from a range of sources is presented in Figure 7.1. These examples, many of which are already in operation in schools, illustrate the scope the school has in promoting physical activity.

Clearly each school has unique characteristics, and the model is intended to be used flexibly and as a stimulus for action, and to help schools to prioritize, plan, select and guide projects and initiatives which are the most feasible and appropriate for them (Cale, 1997).

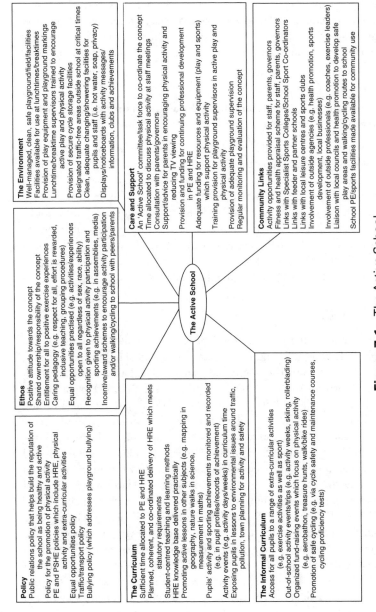

Figure 7.1 The Active School

Source: Adapted and developed from Cale (1997). Reproduced with permission.

Furthermore, a range of specific strategies and initiatives have emanated from government policy (such as the PE, School Sport and Club Links Strategy), and/or been developed by commercial organizations or charitable trusts in recent years which will support schools in the promotion of physical activity and in their quest to become Active Schools (see Chapter 10 for details).

Issues and considerations for schools in promoting physical activity

From the above, it would seem that there have been a number of positive developments concerning the promotion of physical activity in schools and that there is great scope for schools to promote physical activity both within the curriculum and beyond. However, despite such developments and opportunities, it has been suggested that schools may not be maximizing their potential in terms of fostering lifelong activity in youth and that PE could be doing more (Douthitt & Harvey, 1995; Harris & Cale, 1998). Some possible reasons and important issues concerning the promotion of physical activity in schools are explored below.

Status and time

The time allocated to PE in the UK has consistently been among the lowest in Europe and concern regarding the potential health consequences of this has frequently been expressed (Harris, 1994; Fairclough & Stratton, 1997; Morrow, Jackson & Payne, 1999; Cale, 2000a; Fox & Harris, 2003). Fox & Harris (2003) claim that, regrettably, PSHE and PE are generally seen as curricular activities competing with the core subjects of mathematics, English, and science and how, under times of high academic priority, the health and PE curriculum, school sport and therefore physical activity promotion are seen as expendable. Following an international survey of the state and status of PE in schools, Hardman & Marshall (2000) similarly highlighted issues of restricted or decreasing curriculum time for PE, subject status and the attitudes of headteachers, other teachers and parents towards PE. More encouragingly, however, the government's PE, School Sport and Club Links Strategy aims to increase the percentage of schoolchildren in England who spend a minimum of two hours each week in high-quality PE and school sport within and beyond the curriculum from 25 per cent in 2002 to 75 per cent by 2006 (DfES, 2003).

Yet even within existing PE time it seems that physical activity promotion is often not given the time and status it deserves (Cale, 2000a), and there is no guarantee that the situation will change even with additional time. Fox & Harris (2003) highlight how, despite a stronger positioning of health issues within the curriculum in recent years, there is a belief that the effect may be minimal because many teachers prefer to focus on competitive sport in the curriculum.

Teacher knowledge, understanding and attitudes

Many of the concerns over the inconsistent and limited approach, and variations in interpretation, approach and delivery of HRE have been attributed to teachers' lack of knowledge (Harris, 1995; OFSTED, 1996; Cale, Harris & Leggett, 2002). Furthermore, despite PE teachers generally having positive attitudes towards physical activity promotion and/or physical activity and fitness goals (Cale, 2000b; Kulinna & Silverman, 2000) they have been found to have limited physical activity promotion knowledge (Cale, 2000b). Cardon & De Bourdeaudhuij (2002), for example, revealed that many PE teachers were not sufficiently aware of the health-promoting role of PE, and Cale (2000b) reported that a number had a narrow view and limited understanding of the concept of physical activity promotion and how it could be approached in their school.

The above may in part be explained by the fact that few physical educators have been adequately trained to address health-based work and physical activity promotion (Harris, 1997a; Pate et al., 1999; Cardon & De Bourdeaudhuij, 2002; Fox & Harris, 2003). Concerning the preparation of PE teachers in the UK, Fox & Harris (2003) suggest that the structure of courses, as well as financial and time constraints, often afford prospective teachers limited practical exercise teaching experience, which poses problems for the future development of a health-related activity focus. Similarly, the approach many PE teachers adopt to the area has been criticized and blamed on the highly scientized PE/sports science courses (which typically focus on a biophysical conception of the body and of health) from which PE teachers normally graduate (Colquhoun, 1994).

Clearly, the 'subject knowledge' issue needs to be tackled so that teachers feel themselves to be confident and knowledgeable promoters of health and exercise. The Guidance Material published by Harris (2000) is a significant development in this respect. Indeed, a recent study conducted with 500 secondary schools revealed that the material has already had a positive impact on many PE teachers' knowledge, attitudes and confidence, and on their planning, content, evaluation, organization and delivery of HRE (Cale, Harris & Leggett, 2002).

Research developments

During the past decade in particular, a number of advancements in research have bettered our understanding of young people's physical activity and health. Such developments are exciting and welcomed, but they further complicate and have implications for the promotion of physical activity in young people, and teachers clearly need to keep informed and up-to-date. A summary of some of the more relevant recent developments is presented below.

Physical activity guidelines

A major issue in promoting physical activity relates to the type and volume of physical activity young people should be encouraged to do. In order to give young people appropriate exercise guidance, PE teachers clearly need to be aware of the recent exercise recommendations for young people, and their implications for practice, as well as their limitations (Cale & Harris, 1993; 1996). Chapter 5 addresses these issues and provides ideas as to how guidelines can be implemented by physical educators.

The nature of physical activity in children

Researchers have begun to provide a more detailed insight into the nature of young people's physical activity behaviour (e.g. Bailey et al., 1995; Rowland, 1998) (see Chapter 2). Quite simply, children 'do activity in different ways than adults' (Corbin, 2002, p. 132). Fox & Harris (2003) describe young children's activity to involve short, brisk bursts of 'kiss-and-chase' or 'kick-and-run'-type activities and teenagers' activity to be more adult-like and likely to involve sustained moderate activity that is produced through sports or exercise such as jogging or aerobic dance.

Another consideration concerning the nature of young people's activity is the settings in which young people are typically active. Fox & Harris (2003, p. 187) suggest that young people's activity occurs in a range of settings, in a variety of modes and at particular times of the day, and includes:

- active transport to and from school (e.g. walking);
- informal play during school breaks and lunchtimes;
- informal play after school;
- formal sports, PE and exercise training;
- active jobs (for older children).

In recognition that the balance between these modes of being active varies markedly between individuals, and that activity targets can be achieved in very different ways, Fox & Harris (2003) suggest that it may be useful for schools to consider activity profiles in young people. For example, two equally active youngsters in terms of volume of activity might demonstrate very different activity patterns and derive their activity in very different ways. One child may take part in formal sport whereas another may be active through informal play, cycling to school and completing a daily paper round.

The determinants of physical activity in young people
Additionally, knowledge of the determinants of physical activity or reasons why young people do or do not engage in physical activity is important so that teachers can address these factors, challenge the constraints (whether behavioural, social or environmental) to participation and explore with young people ways of overcoming them. The determinants or correlates of young people's physical activity behaviour are considered in detail in Chapter 4.

Making physical activity and sport relevant and attractive to young people

As highlighted earlier, PE time alone cannot satisfy the physical activity needs of young people. It is therefore necessary to consider how PE can most effectively contribute to promoting active lifestyles and provide opportunities for all pupils to experience appropriate levels of physical activity (Cardon & De Bourdeaudhuij, 2002). According to Vilhjalmsson & Thorlindsson (1998), schools primarily affect leisure-time physical activity through positive PE experiences and sport- and exercise-related instruction. Given this, the content and delivery of the PE programme, as well as opportunities within and beyond the school, need to be carefully considered.

In terms of delivery, the desirable practices and principles for the delivery of HRE advocated earlier (Harris, 2000) should be adopted and physical activity promotion needs to be acknowledged as a distinct objective within a structured PE programme. Some specific yet commonly debated issues concerning delivery which are likely to influence young people's experiences and enjoyment of PE include increasing physical activity levels during lessons and fitness testing. Firstly, concerns have been expressed over the low level of moderate-to-vigorous physical activity that children experience during PE lessons (Curtner-Smith, Chen & Kerr, 1995; Stratton, 1996; 1997; Babiarz, Curtner-Smith & Lacon, 1998; Fairclough, 2003). As Chapter 10 reveals, intervention studies have successfully shown that PE can be made more active for pupils, and teachers can make a difference to the amount of activity achieved during lessons (e.g. Simons-Morton et al., 1991; McKenzie et al., 1996; 1997; Sallis et al., 1997; Baquet et al., 2000). Although this is desirable in terms of health benefits and potential pupil involvement and enjoyment, attempts to increase activity need to be approached sensibly. Harris & Cale (1998) caution how increasing activity levels within PE prompts a range of potential responses, some of which may be considered mis-guided and less than desirable. For example, some teachers may respond by adopting a hard-line approach and forcing pupils into 'hard' exercise, such as arduous cross-country running or fitness testing, at the expense of imparting knowledge and understanding about physical activity and developing physical and behavioural skills and positive attitudes towards physical activity. Likewise, Fairclough (2003) suggests that by employing interventions and activities aimed to increase pupils' heart rates (e.g. Baquet, Berthoin & Van Praagh 2002), other teaching objectives within PE may be compromised. According to Cale & Harris (1998), such examples serve only to simplify the complex nature of physical activity promotion and overlook the multifaceted nature of exercise education.

Secondly, fitness testing is common practice in schools (Harris, 1995; ACSM, 2000; Cale & Harris, 2002), yet its value and place in the curri-culum has been widely debated in recent years (Armstrong, 1987; 1989; ACSM, 1988; PEA, 1988; Rowland, 1995; Harris & Cale, 1997; Harris, 2000; Cale & Harris, 2002). The issue of fitness testing is explored in detail in Chapter 9. Suffice it to say here, though, that a potential con-cern with testing in PE lessons is the amount of time spent on it without necessarily positively influencing either pupils' activity levels or their attitudes towards physical activity (Harris & Cale, 1997; Cale & Harris, 2002). Indeed, Rowland (1995) considers programmes of field testing children to be antiethical to the goal of promoting physical activity in children, demeaning, embarrassing and uncomfortable for those children about which there is most concern, and it reinforces the notion that exercise is competitive and unpleasant.

On the issue of the content of the PE curriculum in the UK, Green (2002) and Penney & Evans (1999) have observed that both teachers and government appear to view sport, and particularly team games, as the primary focus of PE and the primary vehicle for the promotion of on-going involvement in health-promoting, active lifestyles. Certainly, despite successive revisions of the NCPE and notwithstanding the loosening of the constraints surrounding games at Key Stage 4 within Curriculum 2000 (DfE & WO, 1995; DfEE & QCA, 1999a), competitive sports and team games with an emphasis on performance still dominate the curriculum (Penney & Harris, 1997; Penney & Evans, 1999; Fairclough, Stratton & Baldwin, 2002). In addition, changes in the terminology towards 'fitness' and 'training', evident within the new requirements (DfEE & QCA, 1999b), further highlight the continued and powerful influence of the focus on sport and performance in PE (Penney & Evans, 1997; 1999; Hargreaves, 2000).

However, the relevance and appeal of competitive sports and team games to many youngsters in the UK has been questioned (Roberts, 1996a; Fairclough, Stratton & Baldwin, 2002; Green 2002; Fox & Harris, 2003) and concern has been expressed that the continued emphasis and privileging of 'traditional PE' may in fact be turning many young people off physical activity participation (Roberts, 1996a; Harris & Cale, 1998; Fox & Harris, 2003). Green (2002), critical of recent government policy in this regard, suggests that much official and semi-official rhetoric concerning school sport and PE fails to acknowledge participatory trends in young people towards lifestyle activities and non-competitive, more recreational sporting forms and away from competitive performance-oriented sports. In so doing, he suggests, it does a substantial disservice to those engaged in PE with a view to promoting lifelong participation by proposing an inappropriate response. Likewise in the US, Douthitt and Harvey (1995, p. 34) are of the opinion that the PE profession has 'been trying to force youth into a PE curriculum mold which does not include sensitivity to individual psycho-emotional needs and preferences'.

On a more positive note, however, Roberts (1996b) and Green (2002) do acknowledge that schools and teachers have begun to respond to the changing lifestyles and activity interests of young people and that the traditional PE diet has now been supplemented by a broader range of activities. If teachers are serious about promoting lifelong physical activity, then this trend needs to continue.

Finally, in response to concerns that the traditional PE programme is neither relevant nor appealing to a large proportion of young people, and taking into account psychosocial factors influencing young people's participation, Fox & Harris (2003) identified a number of features which, in their view, might produce more successful programmes. Features included, for example, introducing more individual sports (e.g. racket, orienteering) and individualized fitness activities (e.g. aerobics, circuits, swimming for fitness); providing activities acceptable to a range of adolescent subcultures (e.g. aerobics, step or aquafit may be more acceptable to girls than hockey or netball); teaching the 'why' of physical activity in the curriculum; helping youngsters to develop self-management skills that equip them to make lifestyle changes; and creating a teaching or coaching climate where children can develop a sense of responsibility.

Discussion point   What is your experience of PE and physical activity promotion in schools?

Based on your experiences, do you feel the issues and concerns highlighted are justified? More specifically:

- Is PE and physical activity promotion afforded status and time?
- Are teachers knowledgeable and positive about physical activity promotion?
- How can teachers keep up to date with relevant research and developments?
- Is the PE programme (content) relevant and attractive for all pupils?
- Is the way in which the PE programme is delivered conducive to promoting physical activity amongst all pupils?

Recommendations

In recent years, several recommendations to direct and guide physical activity promotion within schools have been published in the UK (HEA, 1998; Harris, 2000; National Audit Office, 2001; National Heart Forum, 2002) and in the USA (Centers for Disease Control & Prevention, 1997; 2000; Morrow, Jackson & Payne, 1999). Not surprisingly, these recommendations share many common themes. In particular they identify the need for a whole-school approach to physical activity promotion, targeted physical activity interventions and further research into school-based approaches to promote physical activity.

In analysing the various recommendations, Fox & Harris (2003, p.197) summarize that a whole-school approach to physical activity promotion needs to incorporate the following:

- The development of school policies that promote lifelong physical activity.
- The provision of social and physical environments at school and in the local community that encourage and enable safe and enjoyable physical activity.
- Frequent access to high quality, adequately resourced PE designed to promote physical activity and delivered by appropriately trained and supported staff.
- The promotion of classroom health education that complements physical education.
- The expansion of inclusive extra-curricular programmes that feature a selection of competitive and non-competitive, structured and unstructured, team and individual activities that meet the needs and interests of young people with a wide range of abilities.
- Access to community physical activity programmes that meet the needs and interests of all young people.
- Training for individuals who can play a role in promoting physical activity in young people to help them provide developmentally appropriate, safe and enjoyable activity experiences.
- Parental education and involvement to support school and community programmes that directly support their children's physical activity.

When promoting physical activity, it is also important to realize that the school population is not a homogenous group and targeted interventions are therefore needed. In particular, recommendations highlight the need to target particularly needy populations. For example, within their policy framework, *Young and Active?*, the HEA (1998) calls for interventions differentiated on the grounds of gender, age/life-stage and socio-economic status, and identify girls aged 12–18 years, young people of low socio-economic status and older adolescents as priority groups. Similarly, the President's Council on Physical Fitness and Sports (Morrow, Jackson & Payne, 1999) has called for separate strategies for different age groups formulated around recognized age-specific determinants.

In terms of recommendations for further research, whilst much progress has been made in the area of children's exercise and health generally in recent years, relatively little systematic research has been

undertaken on the effectiveness of school-based approaches to the promotion of young people's physical activity, particularly in the UK and
mainland Europe (Harris & Cale, 1997; Almond & Harris, 1998; Fox &
Harris, 2003). Many school-based interventions have been undertaken
and these are reviewed in Chapter 10. However, and as Chapter 10
illustrates, a lack of rigorous research evaluation has meant that there
has been little opportunity to build an evidence base regarding programme
effectiveness and successful mechanisms for change. Consequently, no
definitive guidelines are available for schools outlining which types of
programmes and strategies are most successful and why. Fox & Harris
(2003) suggest that until such an evidence base is constructed, the design
and delivery of effective activity promotion initiatives will remain uninformed, undirected and sporadic.

Conclusions

Evidently there has been much progress and a number of positive developments concerning physical activity promotion in schools in recent years.
The curriculum, via PE and PSHE, is certainly an important avenue
through which to foster and encourage lifelong participation, and in the
UK the HRE Guidance Material produced by Harris (2000) indicates
significant progress and scope for future improvements in the field.
However, the curriculum is likely to be limited in what it can achieve
without support from the school as a whole. A whole-school approach
to physical activity promotion which focuses on making all aspects of the
school environment conducive to physical activity participation is therefore recommended. Initiatives such as the Healthy Schools Programme
and strategies outlined within the Active School model, as well as a range of
other key initiatives (e.g. those being implemented as part of the PE, School
Sport and Club Links Strategy) and resources (see Chapter 10), are now
attracting increased interest and offer ideas and support to schools.

Despite the developments and opportunities, though, it is suggested
that schools may not be maximizing their potential in terms of fostering
lifelong activity habits, and a number of issues and considerations remain
for schools. For example, issues concerning the status and time afforded
to physical activity promotion, teachers' knowledge, attitudes and confidence in promoting physical activity, the developing research knowledge
base, the relevance and attractiveness of the content and the delivery of
PE and physical activity in schools are all significant. Indeed, it is argued
that, far from promoting physical activity, some developments and

responses to calls for schools to promote physical activity may be misguided and inappropriate, and may therefore be dissuading many young people from participating.

For physical activity promotion to be effective, schools clearly need to address such issues, keep abreast of developments, and provide a committed, consistent, co-ordinated and appropriate approach to physical activity promotion, and clear and consistent messages to young people about physical activity. This may entail questioning, challenging and changing current policies and practices, and will demand a united and concerted effort from all involved.

References

ACCAC (2000a) *Physical Education in the National Curriculum for Wales*. Cardiff: ACCAC.

ACCAC (2000b) *Personal and Social Education Framework. Key Stage 1 to 4 in Wales*. Cardiff: ACCAC.

ACSM (American College of Sports Medicine) (1988) Opinion statement on physical fitness in children and youth, *Medicine and Science in Sport and Exercise*, **20 (4)**, 422–3.

ACSM (American College of Sports Medicine) (2000) Exercise testing and prescription for children, the elderly, and pregnant women. In *ACSM's Guidelines for Exercise Testing and Prescription*, 6th edn. Phildelphia, PA: Lippincott Williams & Wilkins, 217–34.

Almond, L. (1989) New wine in a new bottle – implications for a national physical education curriculum, *The British Journal of Physical Education*, **20(3)**, 123–5.

Almond, L. & Harris, J. (1997) Does health related exercise deserve a hammering or help? *The British Journal of Physical Education*, **28(2)**, 25–7.

Almond, L. & Harris, J. (1998) Interventions to promote health-related physical education. In Biddle, S., Sallis, J. & Cavill, N. (eds), *Young and Active? Young People and Health-Enhancing Physical Activity – Evidence and Implications*. London: HEA, 133–49.

Armstrong, N. (1987) A critique of fitness testing. In Biddle, S. (ed.), *Foundations of Health Related Fitness in Physical Education*. London: Ling Publishing House, 19–27.

Armstrong, N. (1989) Is fitness testing either valid or useful? *British Journal of Physical Education*, **20**, 66–7.

Armstrong, N. (2002) Promoting physical activity and health in youth: the active school and physical education. Abstract presented at the 12th Commonwealth International Sport Conference, 19–23 July, 2002. Manchester, Association of Commonwealth Universities, 37–40.

Babiarz, B., Curtner-Smith, M. D. & Lacon, S. A. (1998) Influence of national curriculum physical education on the teaching of health-related exercise: a case study in an urban setting, *Journal of Sport Pedagogy*, **4**, 1–18.

Bailey, R. C., Olson, J., Pepper, S. L., Porszaz, J., Barstow, T. L. & Cooper, D. M. (1995) The level and tempo of children's physical activities: an observation study, *Medicine and Science in Sports and Exercise*, **27**, 1033–41.

Baquet, G., Berthoin, S. & Van Praagh, E. (2002) Are intensified physical education sessions able to elicit heart rate at a sufficient level to promote aerobic fitness in adolescents? *Research Quarterly for Exercise and Sport*, **73(3)**, 282–8.

Biddle, S. (1991) Promoting health related physical activity in schools. In Armstrong, N. & Sparkes, A. (eds), *Issues in Physical Education*. London: Cassell, 155–69.

Cale, L. (1996) Health related exercise in schools – PE has much to be proud of! *The British Journal of Physical Education*, **27(4)**, 8–13.

Cale, L. (1997) Promoting physical activity through the active school, *The British Journal of Physical Education*, **28(1)**, 19–21.

Cale, L. (2000a) Physical activity promotion in secondary schools, *European Physical Education Review*, **6(1)**, 71–90.

Cale, L. (2000b) Physical activity promotion in schools – PE teachers' views, *European Journal of Physical Education*, **5(2)**, 158–67.

Cale, L. & Harris, J. (1993) Exercise recommendations for children and young people, *Physical Education Review*, **16(2)**, 89–98.

Cale, L. & Harris, J. (1996) Understanding and evaluating the value of exercise guidelines for children. In Lidor, R., Eldar, E. & Harari, I. *Proceedings of the 1995 AIESEP World Congress*, Wingate, Israel, 161–6.

Cale, L. & Harris, J. (1998) The benefits of health-related physical education and recommendations for implementation, *The Bulletin of Physical Education*, **34(1)**, 27–41.

Cale, L. & Harris, J. (2002) National fitness testing for children – issues, concerns and alternatives, *The British Journal of Teaching Physical Education*, **33(1)**, 32–4.

Cale, L., Harris, J. & Leggett, G. (2002) Making a difference? Lessons learned from a health-related exercise resource, *The Bulletin of Physical Education*, **38(3)**, 145–60.

Cardon, G. & De Bourdeaudhuij, I. (2002) Physical education and physical activity in elementary schools in Flanders, *European Journal of Physical Education*, **7(1)**, 5–18.

Centers for Disease Control & Prevention (1997) Guidelines for school and community programs to promote lifelong physical activity among young people, *Morbidity and Mortality Weekly Report*, **46**, RR–6.

Centers for Disease Control & Prevention (2000) *Promoting Better Health for Young People through Physical Activity and Sports*. A report to the President from the Secretary of Health and Human Services and the Secretary of Education.

Colquhoun, D. (1994) Health and physical education in the health promoting school, *Healthy Lifestyles Journal*, **41(1)**, 32.

Corbin, C. B. (2002) Physical activity for everyone: what every physical educator should know about promoting lifelong physical activity, *Journal of Teaching in Physical Education*, **21**, 128–44.

Curtner-Smith, M. D., Chen, W. & Kerr, I. G. (1995) Health-related fitness in secondary school physical education: a descriptive – analytic study, *Educational Studies*, **21(1)**, 55–66.

DES and WO (Department of Education and Science and the Welsh Office) (1992) *Physical Education in the National Curriculum*. London: HMSO.

DCMS (Department for Culture, Media and Sport) (2001) *A Sporting Future for All. The Government's Plan for Sport*. London: DCMS.

DfE and WO (Department for Education and the Welsh Office) (1995) *Physical Education in the National Curriculum*. London: HMSO.

DfEE (Department for Education and Employment) (1997) *Excellence in Schools*. London: HMSO.

DfEE & QCA (Department for Education and Employment & Qualifications and Curriculum Authority) (1999a) *Physical Education. The National Curriculum for England*. London: HMSO.

DfEE & QCA (Department for Education and Employment & Qualifications and Curriculum Authority) (1999b) *The National Curriculum. Handbook for Secondary Teachers in England*. London: HMSO.

DfEE (Department for Education and Skills) (2003) *Learning through PE and Sport. A Guide to the Physical Education, School Sport and Club Links Strategy*. London: DfES.

DoH (Department of Health) (1992) *The Health of the Nation. A Strategy for Health in England*. London: HMSO.

DoH (Department of Health) (1999) *Our Healthier Nation*. London: HMSO.

Douthitt, V. L. & Harvey, M. L. (1995) Exercise counseling – how physical educators can help, *Journal of Physical Education, Recreation and Dance*, **66(5)**, 31–5.

Fairclough, S. (2003) Physical activity lessons during key stage 3 physical education, *The British Journal of Teaching Physical Education*, **34(1)**, 40–5.

Fairclough, S. & Stratton, G. (1997) Physical education curriculum and extra curriculum time: a survey of secondary schools in the North West of England, *The British Journal of Physical Education*, **28(3)**, 21–4.

Fairclough, S., Stratton, G. & Baldwin, G. (2002) The contribution of secondary school physical education to lifetime physical activity, *European Physical Education Review*, **8(1)**, 69–84.

Fox, K. R (1992) Education for exercise and the national curriculum proposals: a step forwards or backwards? *The British Journal of Physical Education*, **23(1)**, 8–11.

Fox, K. (1993) Exercise and the promotion of public health: more messages for the mission, *The British Journal of Physical Education*, **24(3)**, 36–7.

Fox, K. (1996) Physical activity promotion and the active school. In Armstrong, N. (ed.), *New Directions in Physical Education*. London: Cassell Education, 94–109.

Fox, K. & Harris, J. (2003) Promoting physical activity through schools. In McKenna, J. & Riddoch, C. (eds), *Perspectives on Health and Exercise*. Basingstoke: Palgrave Macmillan, 181–201.

Green, K. (2002) Physical education and the 'couch potato society' – part one, *European Journal of Physical Education*, **7(2)**, 95–107.

Hardman, K. & Marshall, J. (2000) The state and status of physical education in the international context, *European Physical Education Review*, **6(3)**, 203–29.

Hargreaves, J. (2000) Gender, morality and the national physical education curriculum. In Hansen, J. & Nielsen, N. (eds), *Sports, Body and Health*. Odense: University Press.

Harris, J. (1994) Physical education in the national curriculum: is there enough time to be effective? *The British Journal of Physical Education*, **25(4)**, 34–8.

Harris, J. (1995) Physical education: a picture of health? *The British Journal of Physical Education*, **26(4)**, 25–32.

Harris, J. (1997a) *Physical Education: A Picture of Health? The Implementation of Health-Related Exercise in the National Curriculum in Secondary Schools in England*. Unpublished doctoral thesis, Loughborough University.

Harris, J. (1997b) A health focus in physical education. In Almond, L. (ed.), *Physical Education in Schools* 2nd edn. London: Kogan Page, 104–20.

Harris, J. (2000) *Health-Related Exercise in the National Curriculum. Key Stages 1 to 4*. Champaign, IL: Human Kinetics.

Harris, J. & Almond, L. (1994) Letter in response to OFSTED inspector's view of HRE in the National Curriculum, *The Bulletin of Physical Education*, **30(3)**, 65–8.

Harris, J. & Cale, L. (1997) How healthy is school PE? A review of the effectiveness of health-related physical education programmes in schools, *Health Education Journal*, **56**, 84–104.

Harris, J. & Cale, L. (1998) Activity promotion in physical education. In Green, K. & Hardman, K. (eds), *Physical Education, A Reader*. Oxford: Meyer & Meyer, 116–31.

Harris, J. & Elbourn, J. (1992) Highlighting health related exercise within the National Curriculum – Part 1, *The British Journal of Physical Education*, **23(1)**, 18–22.

Harris, J. & Penney, D. (2000) Gender issues in health-related exercise, *European Physical Education Review*, **6(3)**, 249–73.

HEA (Health Education Authority) (1998) *Young and Active? Policy Framework for Young People and Health-Enhancing Physical Activity*. London: Author.

Kulinna, P. H. & Silverman, S. (2000) Teachers' attitudes toward teaching physical activity and fitness, *Research Quarterly for Exercise and Sport*, **71(1)**, 80–4.

McBride, N. & Midford, R. (1999) Encouraging schools to promote health: impact of the western Australian school health project (1992–1995), *Journal of School Health*, **69(6)**, 220–5.

McKenzie, G. (2001) Physical activity and health: school interventions. Abstracts of the 6th Annual Congress of the European College of Sports Science, 24–28 July, 17.

McKenzie, T. L., Nader, P. R., Strikmiller, P. K., Yang, M., Stone, E., Perry, C. L. et al. (1996) School physical education: effect of the child and adolescent trial for cardiovascular health, *Preventive Medicine*, **25**, 423–31.

McKenzie, T. L., Sallis, J. F., Kolody, B. & Faucett, F. N. (1997) Long-term effects of a physical education curriculum and staff development work: SPARK, *Research Quarterly in Exercise and Sport*, **68**, 280–91.

Morrow, J. R., Jackson, A. W. & Payne, V. G. (1999) Physical activity promotion and school physical education, *President's Council on Physical Fitness and Sports Research Digest*, **3(7)**, 1–7.

National Audit Office. (2001) *Tackling Obesity in England*. London: The Stationery Office.

NCC (National Curriculum Council) (1990) *Curriculum Guidance 5: Health Education*. London: HMSO.

National Heart Forum (2002) *Young@Heart: A Healthy Start for a New Generation*. London: National Heart Forum.

Nutbeam, D. (1992) The health promoting school: closing the gap between theory and practice, *Health Promotion International*, **7(3)**, 151–3.

OFSTED (Office for Standards in Education) (1996) *Subjects and Standards. Issues for School Development Arising from OFSTED Inspection Findings. 1994/95. Key Stages 3 and 4 and Post 16*. London: HMSO.

Oxley, J. (1994) HRE and the National Curriculum – an OFSTED inspector's view, *Bulletin of Physical Education*, **30(2)**, 39.

Pate, R. R., Small, M. L., Ross, J. G., Young, J. C., Flint, K. H. & Warren, C. W. (1999) *School Physical Education. NASPE Speak II Advocacy Kit*, 19–26.

Penney, D. & Evans, J. (1997) Naming the game. Discourse and domination in physical education and sport in England and Wales, *European Physical Education Review*, **3(1)**, 21–32.

Penney, D. & Evans, J. (1999) *Politics, Policy and Practice in Physical Education*. London: E. & F.N. Spon.

Penney, D. & Harris, J. (1997) Extra-curricular physical education: more of the same for the more able, *Sport, Education and Society*, **2(1)**, 41–54.

PEA (Physical Education Association) (1988) Health related fitness testing and monitoring in schools. A position statement on behalf of the PEA by its Fitness and Health Advisory Committee, *The British Journal of Physical Education*, **19(4/5)**, 194–5.

Roberts, K. (1996a) Young people, schools, sport and government policy, *Sport, Education and Society*, **1(1)**, 47–57.

Roberts, K. (1996b) Youth cultures and sport: the success of school and community sport provisions in Britain, *European Physical Education Review*, **2(2)**, 105–15.

Rowland, T. W. (1995) The horse is dead; let's dismount, *Pediatric Exercise Science*, **7**, 117–20.

Rowland, T. W. (1998) The biological basis of physical activity, *Medicine and Science in Sports and Exercise*, **30**, 392–9.

Sallis, J. F., Bauman, A. & Pratt, M. (1998) Environmental and policy interventions to promote physical activity, *American Journal of Preventive Medicine*, **15(4)**, 379–97.

Sallis, J. F., McKenzie, T. L., Alcaraz, J. E., Kolody, B., Faucette, N. & Hovell, M. F. (1997) The effects of a 2 year physical education programme (SPARK) on physical activity and fitness in elementary school students. Sports, play and active recreation for kids, *American Journal of Public Health*, **87**, 1328–34.

Sallis, J. F. & Owen, N. (1999) *Physical Activity & Behavioural Medicine*. London: Sage.

Shephard, R. J. & Trudeau, F. (2000) The legacy of physical education: influences on adult lifestyle, *Pediatric Exercise Science*, **12**, 34–50.

Simons-Morton, B. G., Parcel, G. S., Baranowski, T., Forthofer, R. & O'Hara, N. M. (1991) Promoting physical activity and a healthful diet among children: results of a school-based intervention study, *American Journal of Public Health*, **81**, 896–991.

Sleap, M. (1990) Promoting health in primary school physical education. In Armstrong, N. (ed.), *New Directions in Physical Education Volume 1*. Champaign, IL: Human Kinetics, 17–36.

Smith, R. A. & Biddle, S. J. H. (1995) Psychological factors in the promotion of physical activity. In Biddle S. J. H. (ed.), *European Perspectives on Exercise and Sport Psychology*. Champaign, IL: Human Kinetics, 85–108.

Stone, E. J., McKenzie, T. L., Welk, G. J. & Booth, M. L. (1998) Effects of physical activity interventions in youth: review and synthesis, *American Journal of Preventive Medicine*, **15(4)**, 298–315.

Stratton, G. (1996) Children's heart rates during physical education lessons: a review, *Pediatric Exercise Science*, **8**, 215–33.

Stratton, G. (1997) Children's heart rates during British physical education lessons, *Journal of Teaching in Physical Education*, **16**, 357–67.

Stratton, G. (1998) Repetition in health related exercise and physical education: mindless or mindful activity? *The British Journal of Physical Education*, **29(4)**, 35–7.

Tones, K. & Tilford, S. (1994) *Health Education. Effectiveness, Efficiency and Equity*, 2nd edn. London: Chapman & Hall.

Vilhjalmsson, R. & Thorlindsson, T. (1998) Factors related to physical activity: a study of adolescents, *Social Science and Medicine*, **47**, 665–75.

Williams, A. (1988) The historiography of health and fitness in physical education, *British Journal of Physical Education Research Supplement*, **3**, 1–4.

Wired for Health (2003) www.wiredforhealth.gov.uk.

8

Promoting Physical Activity within the Community

Chris Riddoch and Jim McKenna

The purpose of this chapter is to explore how 'the community' can influence physical activity opportunities for young people. Essentially, the argument that the community is a powerful influence on how, when, where and how often young people are given the opportunity to be physically active is explored. The primary context of the issue is that many young people are considered to be inactive and, as previously highlighted (see Chapter 2), there are many sound reasons why youngsters should be encouraged to lead an active lifestyle (Blair et al., 1989). This chapter considers the following:

1 The concept of a 'community'.
2 The characteristics of communities that might compromise or promote physical activity in young people.
3 The potentially critical role of the community 'environment'.
4 Community-based initiatives that may enhance young people's activity opportunities.

These issues are not dealt with in isolation, as they are mutually informative. Rather, an argument is presented that places elements of the environment, physical, social and cultural, at the heart of young people's

191

opportunities for (in)activity. Whenever there is a desire to reverse an adverse trend in society (and increasing sedentariness is certainly an undesirable trend), there are a number of ways in which the problem might be tackled. First, individuals might be encouraged to become more active (e.g. activity promotion campaigns). Secondly, individuals might be forced to become more active (e.g. removing sedentary opportunities such as lifts). Thirdly, it could be made very difficult for individuals to maintain inactive habits (e.g. placing a tax on inactive pursuits). Fourthly, individuals could be given individualized programmes for increasing activity change (e.g. exercise-referral schemes), making them aware of the main barriers to active lifestyles and giving them psychological strategies that they can employ to overcome them (e.g. counselling). (See Chapter 6 for an overview of theoretical models of exercise behaviour change.)

All of the above have been tried in the field of health promotion and most of them in the field of physical activity promotion. Most have failed, at least in terms of stimulating long-term change in large numbers of people. This is disappointing, but heart can be taken from the fact that perhaps the most obvious strategy, actually removing the original causes of sedentary living, has not yet been tried. The effects of modifying the environment within which we live, the environment that forces us at almost every turn to choose inactive options, has yet to be evaluated. Largely, this may be because such initiatives are commonly thought to be too difficult and too expensive. However, if population-level change is desired, as opposed to just a few individuals changing for the better, the nettle of removing the true causes must be grasped. In other words, communities must address the issue of exactly why the members of those communities are inactive. In the UK, and probably in the rest of the western world, the reasons almost certainly lie within the types of environment in which most people live.

Communities and inactivity

So what, then, is a community? Communities can be anything that suggests communality, gatherings or networks of people. Communities can be schools, leisure centres, sports clubs, neighbourhoods, households/families, clubs and societies, or friendship groups. Minkler & Wallerstein (1996), cited in Pate et al. (2000, p. 138), have suggested that a community is 'a group of people who share values and institutions. Communities are social groups that operate as a functional spatial unit, a unit of patterned social interaction, or a symbolic unit of collective identity.' The authors further suggest that community interventions to promote health-enhancing behaviour combine organizing the community and involving citizens with strategies of lifestyle, policy and/or environmental interventions.

And what is the community's 'environment'? This is important as there is agreement that the root cause of inactivity is our physical environment and the changes that have taken place since the industrial revolution. Cars, TV and labour-saving devices now abound and each one reduces personal activity by considerable amounts. The great majority of people today have sedentary occupations. Schooling, which occupies the majority of young people's time, is essentially a 'sitting down' experience. It might also be argued that our social environment with respect to physical activity has also changed for the worse. For example, many TV adverts promote their wares by suggesting that they are 'labour-saving' ('it's less bovver with a hover', a TV advert for a mechanized lawnmower which shows a man asleep in a hammock instead of pushing the mower.)

Pate et al. (2000) claim that community-level interventions may be critical for young people, as they spend large amounts of time in community settings. Indeed, all the communities suggested (e.g. schools, leisure centres, sports clubs, etc.) can have a unique effect on young people's attitudes towards and participation in physical activity. It would be possible to investigate each one in terms of its influence, cultural importance and current role. However, such an analysis would necessarily be superficial, as little research has been conducted concerning their specific effects on young people's activity (see Chapter 10). Suffice it to say that they are probably all important and all have undoubted roles to play in any initiative to foster healthier activity levels in young people. The important issue may be not to look at them in isolation, but rather to consider that they all operate in a physical, social and cultural environment that determines how effective young people are.

The central issue is that any physical activity improvement initiative which focuses on individuals, whether community-based or not, is unlikely to have any marked effect if it operates within an environment that is toxic to physical activity. Individuals may be motivated to become more active within such initiatives, and even make the initial steps towards increasing their activity, but once these individuals are released back into the environment, the original pressures to be sedentary immediately confront them. It is the contention of this chapter that these pressures to be sedentary defeat all but a few psychologically strong individuals. Mostly, people succumb to the sedentary pressures that surround them in their communities. They may continue to take regular 'shelter' within, for example, an exercise class or sports club, but this may only provide temporary, albeit welcome, relief from sedentary living. Essentially, their days are still filled with sedentary activities. How these pressures apply to and influence young people, and to what extent young people are 'forced' into sedentary activities, needs to be considered. Chapter 4 considers sedentary behaviours and the correlates of sedentary behaviour in young people, calling for more research in this area.

The essential point to grasp is that it is the changes that have taken place within communities *per se*, especially the physical characteristics of communities, which have caused severe reductions in activity levels. There has been no communal, nationwide population decision to take less exercise. Rather, it has happened surreptitiously, stealthily, without most even noticing. It has happened via the changing nature of work, transport policy, education policy, building design, town planning and a plethora of gadgets, media messages and alternative yet attractive sedentary leisure pursuits. Further, such changes have occurred within just one generation.

Young people are probably not immune to all of this and the potential for population-level change in young people's physical activity must therefore be considered. Population-level change is vital, as this is how meaningful improvements in public health can be achieved. Whereas encouraging individual youngsters to take extra activity will no doubt benefit those youngsters (and this is significant), it is of prime importance to consider how the activity levels of *all* young people can be improved. The strategies that promote activity by focusing on individuals seem to have short-term success but experience long-term failure. In other words, individuals make great efforts to change and become more active, but the effort involved (in terms of time, planning, facilities, cost, etc.) is too great to maintain long-term. The inexorable pressures to be sedentary emanating from the physical make-up of the community eventually defeat even the steeliest resolve to be more active. This is not true for everybody, of course. Some people do manage to maintain an active lifestyle long-term and these individuals might indeed constitute an important population for future research. Nevertheless, the great majority revert to sedentary living eventually. In the same vein, individuals who lose weight tend mostly to regain it. Thus, it may be the community that can have the greatest influence, as it is the local community that takes responsibility for the local environment.

Activity

Consider the characteristics of your community that might compromise or promote physical activity in young people. Conduct a SWOT analysis (i.e. identify the strengths, weaknesses, opportunities and threats to young people's physical activity participation) to determine how conducive your community is or could be to physical activity? For example, your community may have:

- a Specialist Sports College (strength)
- limited open (and safe) spaces to play (weakness)
- plans to build a new leisure centre (opportunity)
- a large shopping centre which attracts youngsters after school and at weekends (threat).

Causes of inactivity in young people

It has been known for some time that young people's freedom to be active has been endangered. Hillman (1993) reported that between 1971 and 1990 there had been marked reductions in walking to school, low levels of cycling to school (from 80 per cent to 9 per cent), and generally less licence offered to children by their parents to play out on their own and be independent. Recent surveys (Joint Health Surveys Unit, 1998; Gregory & Lowe, 2000) have confirmed these trends and the general view is that many children are now insufficiently active for optimal health benefit (see Chapter 2). As highlighted in Chapter 2, the National Diet and Nutrition Survey indicated that approximately 40 per cent of boys and 60 per cent of girls did not achieve recommended levels of physical activity (i.e. on average one hour of moderate physical activity per day) (Gregory & Lowe, 2000). Girls are less active than boys, especially after adolescence, and both boys and girls become less active as they get older. Furthermore, the British Heart Foundation (2000) reveal that over 25 per cent of 11–16-year-olds watch more than four hours of television per day and that physical education in primary schools has more than halved over a five-year period.

Whether the environment is indeed the cause of such worrying changes/trends warrants investigation. To date, environmental barriers to and determinants of physical activity have largely been investigated in adults. In these studies, poor weather has been reported to be a barrier (Sallis et al., 1999). Also, individuals living in coastal (Bauman et al., 1999) or rural rather than suburban or inner-city areas (Potvin et al., 1997) are more likely to engage in physical activity. In rural communities, physically demanding occupations and easier access to active leisure pursuits are predictors of activity (Potvin et al., 1997). Among older adults, access to footpaths and local parks are associated with increased levels of walking (Booth et al., 2000). Access to walking trails has also been reported to be important, and trails have been found to be particularly beneficial in encouraging physical activity amongst segments of the population at highest risk of inactivity, for example women and individuals in lower socio-economic groups (Brownson et al., 2000). Further, safe and convenient facilities for walking have predicted higher levels of regular walking in both women and men (Owen et al., 2000). Other significant factors include scenery (King et al., 2000) and safety, particularly for women (Pinto et al., 1996) and ethnic minority youths (Garcia et al., 1995).

Access to environmental physical activity facilities have also been shown to be predictive of physical activity levels, again especially in women (Rutten et al., 2001). In a study of street layouts in the United States (human transit-oriented versus car-oriented), it was found that more pedestrian activity occurred where street design was oriented to the human rather than the car (Cervero Gorham, 1995). 'Neighbourhoods without neighbours' is a term used to describe situations where people who live next to each other and are close spatially actually remain isolated from one another in other respects. Finally, in a study utilizing Geographic Information Systems (GIS) in a busy street, travel distance to access the facility and hilly terrain were found to be barriers to the use of a community rail-trail (Troped et al., 2001).

Despite the limited research on the influence of environmental factors on young people's physical activity, consistent associations have nonetheless been reported (Sallis, Prochaska & Taylor, 2000) (see Chapter 4). As Chapter 4 acknowledges, access to facilities and programmes and time spent outside are associated with greater physical activity in young people.

Natural activities of young people

One major change that seems to have taken place is that young people today spend less time outdoors during their free time and conversely spend more time involved in indoor, more sedentary activities. There is evidence to suggest that young people are now living in an increasingly physically restricted environment, especially in urban areas. Indeed, in some ways it could be argued that children are being kept under something akin to 'house arrest'. As has just been highlighted, time spent outdoors is known to be associated with overall physical activity in children, but parents may restrict their children's time outdoors because appropriate and safe places are perceived not to be available (Sallis, 1993). Although the fears of parents are entirely understandable and to be expected, the challenge is to remove the causes of those fears and perceptions that lead to possibly an overconcern for child safety.

Aside from parental restrictions as a consequence of concerns over safety, it seems that adults generally are imposing restrictions on young people's activity. For example, *The Times* of 6 August 2003 carried an article entitled 'Killjoy adults stop children's outdoor play', in which it was reported that 80 per cent of children have been told off for playing on the streets, on estates and in parks. Britain was described as in danger of becoming a 'child free zone' as children are increasingly 'tidied away'. Such actions probably deny children their right to play, as enshrined in the Human Rights Act 1998 and the UN Convention on the Rights of the Child, and undoubtedly constrain their opportunities to be active.

Hillman (http://www.spokeseastkent.org.uk/mayer.htm) has spoken of our current fears for children when they venture independently into the community. He cites numerous examples, including the 'walking bus', whereby children and parents appear to pick their way through an apparent minefield on their way to school, 'safe houses' where children are told they can find help if they feel threatened, Parent Watch schemes to supervise children's play, and 'stranger/danger' campaigns that advise children to 'yell, run and tell' if approached by a stranger. Such initiatives are undoubtedly valuable, well-meaning and warranted in some areas, and they may ease the fears of parents and possibly the children, but it is difficult to escape the feeling that such a siege mentality may be somewhat of an overreaction, a possible end result being that young people become 'too safe' to the extent that their physical and cognitive development may be impaired.

Childhood can be conceptualized as both the 'free of worries' stage of life and a particularly vulnerable and/or 'risky' period as well. Parental 'risk perception' could well play a pivotal role in the fostering of physical activity opportunities for young people. Parental concerns about the safety of their children may have become a major contemporary influence on young people's physical activity behaviour. Childhood may have been transformed from a 'reckless' stage of life to an inherently 'risky' period of life. Parents often regulate the boundaries within which childhood is experienced, possibly overregulating it if their perceptions of safety and danger are ill-founded. Of course, this may not always be the case, but it is reasonable to presume that the responsibilities of parenthood have at least partly been transformed from provision of childhood, to provision of protection from the risks of childhood.

Yet parents have probably always been concerned about cars, accidents, abduction and sexual abuse, so any new risks are not necessarily associated with parental perceptions in a deterministic way. In fact, it may not be the dangers *per se* that prevent parents from allowing children to play outside, but rather the lack of supervision and surveillance.

Theoretical aspects

It has been established that communities, especially the physical/environmental make-up of communities, can clearly limit physical activity. The community may therefore offer significant potential for encouraging activity at the population level. Further, because the physical, environmental modifications within the community are relatively permanent, they become part of the physical infrastructure, and any resulting improvements in physical activity will be sustained long-term. Whether community-level interventions are justified theoretically, however, needs to be investigated. It has frequently been shown that public health strategies that are not theoretically based are less likely to be effective, and therefore a theoretical foundation and framework is essential.

A number of authors have argued for an environmental or community-based approach to promoting physical activity, including in young people (Pate et al., 2000; Richter et al., 2000; Sallis et al., 2000) (see also Chapters 4, 7 and 10). Kerr et al. (2002) have postulated that environmental strategies to promote physical activity can be justified from a range of theoretical perspectives including Organizational Development Theory (Dwyer, 1997), Human Ecological Theory (Green et al., 1996), Social Ecological Theory (Stokols, 1992; 1996), Diffusion of Innovations Theory (Schmid et al., 1995) and Behavioural Choice Theory (Epstein, 1998). Considered together, these theoretical frameworks provide a multilayered conceptualization of the environment. Duhl (1996), who describes the environment as a web of biological, spatial, physical, social, political and cultural relationships, reinforces this view. This multidimensional view of the environment is also reflected by Stokols (1992), who defines the physical environment as geographic, architectural and technical, and the social environment as cultural, economical and political.

It is important to note that the above considerations largely view the environment in isolation. However, we know that environmental variables are not the only influences on behaviour (Sallis et alet al., 1998). Rather, there exists a reciprocal and dynamic interaction between individuals and their environment. As a consequence, environmental change must be regarded from a similarly interactive perspective (Sparling et al., 2000). Any community-based initiative must therefore take account of this. Several authors provide examples of such multidimensional models and frameworks for understanding the process of environmental change (Stokols, 1996; Wandersman et al., 1996; Dwyer, 1997; Sallis et al., 1998; Sallis et al., 1999; Swinburn et al., 1999; Owen et al., 2000) and we are now at a stage where a deeper understanding of a complex phenomenon is within reach. Whereas, in the past, community-based, environmental approaches have, owing to their complexity, not been worked out in great detail (Green et al., 1996), or relegated to the 'too-hard basket' (Nutbeam, 1997), there is now a clear justification and need for research in this area (Sallis et al., 1998). The community may provide the key to stimulating meaningful improvements in activity levels in both young people and adults.

The case for community-level intervention

From the preceding sections, it is clear that there exists a theoretical, logistical and empirical justification for evaluating the effectiveness of environmental interventions to promote physical activity. It is known that such changes, should they be achieved, will result in significant improvements in physical, social and psychological health (Riddoch & Boreham, 1999; Department of Health, in press). Community interventions most potently affect habitual 'lifestyle' activities, such as active commuting to work or school, although they also provide opportunities for more active recreation. However, it is the encouragement of habitual lifestyle activities that is likely to be the cornerstone of population change.

With this in mind, habitual walking and cycling are ideal forms of health-related physical activity (Kifer, 2000) and can easily be incorporated into everyday life by both young people and adults. This is especially true of travelling to and from work and school (Oja et al., 1998). In adults, many studies have shown the health benefits to be gained. Walking three miles per week has been associated with a 13 per cent reduction in coronary heart disease events (Sesso et al., 2000) and cycling for one hour or for 25 miles per week has been associated with a 50 per cent reduction in risk of dying from all causes over a ten-year follow-up period (Morris et al., 1990). Cycling to work has also been associated with a 30 per cent lower risk of mortality in both men and women (Andersen et al., 2000). In the Osaka Health Study, walking for 11–20 minutes to work was associated with a 12 per cent reduced risk of incidence of hypertension, and walking for more than 20 minutes was associated with a 29 per cent reduction in risk (Hayashi et al., 1999). Meanwhile, Vuori et al., (1994) have shown that in Finland those individuals who actively commute to work have both higher levels of cardiorespiratory fitness and reduced coronary heart disease risk factors. It is difficult to imagine that these profound health benefits seen in adults are not reflected in important ways in young people who participate in similar types of activities.

The problem is, of course, that over the last half century there has been a dramatic shift, within the developed world, away from walking and cycling as modes of personal transport to a reliance on the car. In the UK, since 1985 the distance individuals travel on foot per year has decreased by 22 per cent and cycling distance has decreased by 10 per cent. Over this same period, mean distance travelled by car has increased by 41 per cent (DETR, 1999). It is precisely this loss of 'lifestyle' physical activity that constitutes the root of the problem. Young people are involved in this, as evidenced by the 'school run'.

Initiating community-level, environmental change

As well as researchers calling for environmental or community-based approaches to the promotion of physical activity, there are an increasing number of calls for initiatives that can be broadly described as 'environmental' from government and other organizations. For example, the National Service Framework for coronary heart disease recommends increased active transport and more Active Schools. The School Travel Advisory Group is investigating the physical environments that surround schools. The Urban White Paper stresses sustainable transport, promotion of pedestrian and cycle access to jobs and shopping, and managing the pattern of urban growth to promote ease of access to facilities. (See Chapters 7 and 10 for further details of some of these initiatives.)

Environmental manipulations can operate at many levels, from the individual level to the global level, and demand a multidisciplinary and multi-agency approach. They also necessitate extensive, structured and systematic collaboration (Wandersman et al., 1996; Harris & Wills, 1997; Kickbusch, 1997). Such large-scale environmental approaches to public health are not new, with many successful initiatives incorporating environmental and/or policy change. Examples include housing sanitation, water purification, water fluoridation and road safety (Schmid et al., 1995; King, 1999). However, such initiatives have yet to be applied and rigorously evaluated in the field of physical activity, largely because of the high costs of restructuring the environment.

Nevertheless, large-scale environmental interventions to promote physical activity do exist. For example, Sustrans (Sustainable Transport) is a well-established organization whose remit is to build and manage a broad range of environmental interventions to promote sustainable transport to school and work, and opportunities for active recreation. One such major initiative is the creation of the National Cycle Network. Such initiatives are highly important, a point made abundantly clear by Lawlor et al., in press): 'environmental interventions aimed at increasing physical activity are public health's best buy. The National Cycle Network (a Sustrans project) represents the UK's largest environmental intervention of this nature.'

Solutions

There may be very positive signs for the future. On 22 May 2003, the Heritage Lottery Fund published research highlighting that children are not necessarily the 'couch potatoes' that we believe them to be. The research reported that children prefer visiting parks to watching TV (at least on a nice day), that the local park is a very important part of their life, and that 95 per cent of young families visit the park regularly. Further, children talk with great emotion about the important role of the park and the activity opportunities it affords in growing up. It may be, therefore, that the natural exuberance of youngsters for physical activity is currently not being channelled. Rather, adults are 'keeping them in the house' because the outside environment is perceived to be either unsafe or unattractive.

As previously stated, Hillman (1993) documented a severe decline in children's freedom to travel independently and a reduction in the number of 'licences' given to children to walk to school over a 20-year period. Generally, the personal freedom and choice permitted a typical seven-year-old in 1971 are now not permitted until children reach the age of about nine and a half. This may be against the natural instincts of the young person. The potential for community-level interventions to improve the environment might be successful in encouraging young people's natural instincts to participate in active pursuits. This might operate directly through the youngsters, or indirectly through changing their parents' perceptions of safety.

If the community is to act as the agent of change, then a flexible, multidisciplinary approach which incorporates interaction between key individuals, organizations and communities may be most appropriate. It is therefore very encouraging that 2004 heralds the release of the Chief Medical Officer's Review of Physical and Health Outcomes (Department of Health, in press), which contains a section on young people within an overall 'lifecourse' perspective. In parallel with this review, is the establishment of a cross-governmental panel, the Activity Co-ordination Team, which monitors the policies of a wide range of government departments (including the Department for Education and Skills; the Department for Transport, Local Government and the Regions; the Department for Culture, Media and Sport; the Department of Health) in terms of how they promote increased physical activity.

The greatest barrier to community-level change may be its complexity. Whereas rewards may be great, persuading corporations and communities to engage in environmental initiatives may be challenging. Examples of community-level change might include tax and other incentives, changes that must be made at the political level. Although the focus here is on young people, the ultimate aim of environmental change should be to facilitate increased activity in all sections of society as this will lead to maximum public health improvement.

A major feature of community-level interventions is that, unlike behavioural and educational approaches, they do not hold individuals responsible for the desired change. This is extremely important because, as mentioned previously, individuals may be able to initiate change successfully, but they cannot themselves maintain the change long-term. Community interventions would promote increased activity via subtle, almost unconscious processes, where failure to change is not a reason for self-blame. To give a simple example, if the only way for individuals to reach the fourth floor of a building is via the stairs, then they take the stairs! Such initiatives are more likely to yield substantial public health dividends and will produce longer-term effects, as the interventions are permanent within the environment. In effect, they become embedded within the community and can create healthy social norms. Thus, taking the stairs becomes a normal not a deviant behaviour.

Resources and guides for action

Specific examples of community-level physical activity interventions are hard to come by. The few that are available are reviewed in Chapter 10. That said, there are many relevant publications that can inform the design and delivery of community-focused interventions. Kerr et al., (2002) propose a useful taxonomy of possible community and environmental strategies. Some constitute low-cost environmental interventions that any community could consider. Others are higher-cost but are still within the remit of most local authorities. The following are a selection of recommended strategies that might be considered relevant to young people:

- pedestrian zones
- green zones
- home zones
- low-cost sports facilities
- parks – lighting, shaded areas, play facilities
- neighbourhood clean-ups for parks, roads and beaches
- separate walkways for pedestrians
- pedestrian-friendly pavements
- link cycle and walking paths to public transport
- link urban routes to countryside
- enable travel by cycling and public transport
- secure cycle-parking facilities
- improve cycle safety
- incorporate cycling in highway management and public transport schemes
- reduce traffic speeds
- restrictions on heavy goods vehicles.

Pate et al. (2000) also offer similar suggestions for young people and include additional options such as easy carriage of bicycles on subways and transit systems, and economic incentives for including physical activity promotion into the design of buildings. Further, they provide a list of factors that can influence the process of instigating community-level change:

- Begin from a base of community ownership of problems and solutions
- Use relevant theory, data and local experiences to systematically plan, implement and evaluate the intervention programme
- Assess what types of intervention are acceptable and feasible for specific populations and circumstances
- Establish an organizational and advocacy programme to orchestrate multiple intervention strategies into a complementary, cohesive programme
- Conduct appropriate evaluation activities during and after the intervention period. (Pate et al., 2000, p. 140)

The American Heart Association has produced a guide for public health practitioners, healthcare providers and health policy makers for improving cardiovascular health at the community level, much of which is relevant to young people. Likewise, the National Centre for Chronic Disease Prevention and Health Promotion publish *Promoting Physical Activity: A Guide for Community Action* and the Congress for the New Urbanism issues a publication that speaks of 'reclaiming our homes, blocks, streets, parks, neighbourhoods, districts, towns, cities, regions and environment' (http://www.cnu.org).

Initiatives such as 'Active Living by Design' (http://www.activeliv-ingbydesign.org), 'ACES' (Active Community Environments Initiative) (http://www.cdc.gov/nccdphp/dnpa/aces/htm) and 'Walkable Communities' are also relevant. 'Active Living by Design' is a national pro-gramme in the United States concerned with innovative approaches to increasing physical activity through community design, public policies and communications strategies. 'ACES' promotes walking, cycling and the development of accessible recreation facilities. To achieve this, data are utilized from a variety of disciplines including public health, urban design and transport planning. This combination of data suggests that characteristics of communities such as proximity of facilities, street design, density of housing, availability of public transit and of pedestrian and bicycle facilities, play an important role in promoting or discour-aging physical activity. 'Walkable Communities' is an organization that considers 'walkability' as the cornerstone and key to an urban area's success (http://www.walkable.org).

Finally, there are also a number of initiatives to foster opportunities for children's play which may be long overdue. For example, 'Zoneparc' is currently being established in schools in the UK. This promotes the development of innovative playground opportunities for children (see Chapter 10 for further details). Further, the New Opportunities Fund has made £200 million available to encourage new children's play opportunities.

Conclusions

Progress is being made concerning the promotion of physical activity within the community. However, there is still much to do. If community approaches are to be truly effective, then community attitudes to young people will need to change, to refocus and re-establish young people as having legal rights to a healthy, active childhood. There must be consideration of young people in all aspects of planning, including transport, building, open spaces and leisure facilities. Only in this way will the health, wellbeing and quality of life of this and future generations of young people be protected.

References

Andersen, L. B., Schnohr, P., Schroll, M. & Hein, H. O. (2000) All-cause mortality associated with physical activity during leisure time, work, sports, and cycling to work, *Archives of Internal Medicine*, **160(11)**, 1621–8.

Bauman, A., Smith, B., Stoker, L., Bellew, B. & Booth, M. L. (1999) Geographical influences upon physical activity participation, evidence of a 'coastal effect', *Australian and New Zealand Journal of Public Health*, **23**, 322–4.

Blair, S. N., Clark, D. G., Cureton, K. J. & Powell, K. E. (1989) Exercise and fitness in childhood: implications for a lifetime of health. In Gisolfi, C. V. & Lamb, D. R. (eds), *Perspectives in Exercise Science and Sports Medicine*, vol. 2: *Youth, Exercise and Sport*. New York: McGraw Hill 401–30.

Booth, M. L., Owen, N., Bauman, A., Clavisi, O. & Leslie, E. (2000) Social-cognitive and perceived environment influences associated with physical activity in older Australians, *Preventive Medicine*, **31(1)**, 15–22.

British Heart Foundation (2000) *Couch Kids – The Growing Epidemic*. London: British Heart Foundation.

Brownson, R. C., Housemann, R. A., Brown, D. R., Jackson-Thompson, J., King, A. C., Malone, B. R. & Sallis, J. F. (2000) Promoting physical activity in rural communities, *American Journal of Preventive Medicine*, **18**, 235–41.

Cervero, R. & Gorham, R. (1995) Commuting in transit versus automobile neighbourhoods, *Journal of the American Planning Association*, **61(2)**, 210–25.

DETR (Department of the Environment, Transport and the Regions) (1999) *Transport Statistics. Transport Trends: Walking and Cycling in Great Britain*. London: DETR.

DoH (Department of Health) (in press) *Physical Activity and Health Outcomes: A Review of the Chief Medical Officer*. London: DoH.

Duhl, L. J. (1996) An ecohistory of health: the role of 'healthy cities', *American Journal of Health Promotion*, **10**, 258–61.

Dwyer, S. (1997) Improving delivery of a health-promoting-environments program: experiences from Queensland Health, *Australian and New Zealand Journal of Public Health*, **21**, 398–402.

Epstein, L. H. (1998) Integrating theoretical approaches to promote physical activity, *American Journal of Preventive Medicine*, **15**, 257–65.

Garcia, A. W., Broda, M. A. N., Frenn, M., Coviak, C., Pender, N. J. & Ronas, D. L. (1995) Gender and developmental differences in exercise beliefs among youth and prediction of their exercise behaviour, *Journal of School Health*, **65**, 213–19.

Green, L. W., Richard, L. & Potvin, L. (1996) Ecological foundations of health promotion, *American Journal of Health Promotion*, **10**, 270–81.

Gregory, J. & Lowe, S. (2000) *National Diet and Nutrition Survey: Young People Aged 4 to 18 Years*. London: The Stationery Office.

Harris, E. & Wills, J. (1997) Developing healthy local communities at local government level: lessons from the past decade, *Australian and New Zealand Journal of Public Health*, **21**, 403–12.

Hayashi, T., Tsumura, K., Suematsu, C., Okada, K., Fijii, S. & Endo, G. (1999) Walking to work and the risk for hypertension in men: the Osaka Health Survey, *Annals of Internal Medicine*, **131(1)**, 21–6.

Hillman, M. (1993) One false move: an overview of the findings and issues they raise. In Hillman, M., *Children, Transport and the Quality of Life*, London: Policy Studies Institute, 7–18.

Joint Health Surveys Unit (1998) *Health Survey for England: The Health of Young People 1995–1997*. London: HMSO.

Kerr, J., Eves, F. & Carroll, D. (2002) The environment: the greatest barrier? In McKenna, J. & Riddoch, C. J. (eds), *Critical Perspectives in Physical Activity and Health*. Basingstoke: Palgrave Macmillan, 203–25.

Kickbusch, I. (1997) Health-promoting environments: the next steps, *Australian and New Zealand Journal of Public Health*, **21**, 431–4.

Kifer, K. (2000) Cycling and health. Why promote cycling? *British Medical Journal*, **321(7257)**, 387.

King, A. C. (1999) Environmental and policy approaches to the promotion of physical activity. In Rippe, J. M. & Norwalk, C. T. (eds), *Lifestyle Medicine*. Oxford: Blackwell Science.

King, A. C., Castro, C., Wilcox, S., Eyler, A. A., Sallis, J. F. & Brownson, R. C. (2000) Personal and environmental factors associated with physical inactivity among different racial–ethnic groups of U. S. middle-aged and older-aged women, *Health Psychology*, **19(4)**, 354–64.

Lawlor, D. A., Ness, A., Cope, A. M., Davis, A., Insall, P. & Riddoch, C. J. (2003). The National Cycle Network: 'Public Health's best buy'? *Journal of Epidemiology & Community Health*, **57**, 96–101.

Morris, J. N., Clayton, D. G., Everitt, M. G., Semmence, A. M. & Burgess, E. H. (1990) Exercise in leisure time: coronary attack and death rates, *British Heart Journal*, **63**, 325–34.

Nutbeam, D. (1997) Creating health-promoting environments: overcoming barriers to action, *Australian and New Zealand Journal of Public Health*, **21**, 355–9.

Oja, P., Vuori, I. & Paronen, O. (1998) Daily walking and cycling to work: their utility as health-enhancing physical activity, *Patient Education and Counseling*, **33**(1 supplement), S87–94.

Owen, N., Leslie, E., Salmon, J. & Fotheringham, M. J. (2000) Environmental determinants of physical activity and sedentary behavior, *Exercise and Sport Science Reviews*, **28(4)**, 153–8.

Pate, R., Trost, S., Mullis, R., Sallis, J., Wechsler, H. & Brown, D. (2000) Community interventions to promote proper nutrition and physical activity among youth, *Preventive Medicine*, **31**, S138–49.

Pinto, B. M., Marcus, B. H. & Clark, M. M. (1996) Promoting physical activity in women: the new challenges, *American Journal of Preventive Medicine*, **12**, 395–400.

Potvin, L., Gauvin, L. & Nguyen, N. M. (1997) Prevalence of stages of change for physical activity in rural, suburban and inner-city communities, *Journal of Community Health*, **22**, 1–13.

Richter, K. P., Harris, K. P., Paine-Andrews, A., Fawcett, S. B., Schmid, T. L., LanKenau, B. H. & Johnston, J. (2000) Measuring the health environment for physical activity and nutrition among youth: a review of the literature and applications for community initiatives, *Preventive Medicine*, **31**(supplement), S98–111.

Riddoch, C. J. & Boreham, C. A. G. (1999) Physical activity, fitness and children's health: current concepts. In Van Mechelen, W. Armstrong, N. (eds), *Paediatric Exercise Science and Medicine*. Oxford: Oxford University Press, 243–52.

Rutten, A., Abel, T., Kannas, L., von Lengerke, T., Luschen, G., Diaz, J. A. R., Vinck, J. & van der Zee, J. (2001) Self reported physical activity, public health, and perceived environment: results from a comparative European study, *Journal of Epidemiology and Community Health*, **55**(2), 139–46.

Sallis, J. F. (1993) Epidemiology of physical activity and fitness in children and adolescents, *Critical Reviews in Food Science and Nutrition*, **33**(4/5), 403–8.

Sallis, J. F., Bauman, A. & Pratt, M. (1998) Environmental and policy interventions to promote physical activity, *American Journal of Preventive Medicine*, **15**(4), 379–97.

Sallis, J. F. & Owen, N. (1999) *Physical Activity and Behavioural Medicine*. Thousand Oaks, CA: Sage, 102–6.

Sallis, J., Patrick, K., Frank, E., Pratt, M., Wechsler, H. & Galuska, D. (2000) Interventions in healthcare settings to promote healthful eating and physical activity in children and adolescents, *Preventive Medicine*, **31**(supplement), S112–20.

Sallis, J., Prochaska, J. & Taylor, W. (2000) A review of correlates of physical activity of children and adolescents, *Medicine and Science in Sports and Exercise*, **32**, 963–75.

Schmid, T. L., Pratt, M. & Howze, E. (1995) Policy as intervention: Environmental and policy approaches to the prevention of cardiovascular diseases, *American Journal of Public Health*, **85**, 1207–11.

Sesso, H. D., Paffenbarger, R. S. Jr. & Lee, I. M. (2000) Physical activity and coronary heart disease in men: The Harvard Alumni Health Study, *Circulation*, **102**(9), 975–80.

Sparling, P., Owen, O., Lambert, E. V. & Haskell, W. L. (2000) Promoting physical activity: the new imperative for public health, *Health Education Research*, **15**, 367–76.

Stokols, D. (1992) Establishing and maintaining healthy environments: toward a social ecology of health promotion, *American Psychologist*, **47**, 6–22.

Stokols, D. (1996) Translating social ecological theory into guidelines for community health promotion, *American Journal of Health Promotion*, **10**, 282–98.

Swinburn, B., Egger, G. & Raza, F. (1999) Dissecting obesogenic environments: The development and application of a framework for identifying and prioritizing environmental interventions for obesity, *Preventive Medicine*, **29**, 563–70.

Troped, P. J., Saunders, R. P., Pate, R. R., Reininger, B., Ureda, J. R. & Thompson, S. J. (2001) Associations between self-reported and objective physical environmental factors and use of a community rail-trail, *Preventive Medicine*, **32(2)**, 191–200.

Vuori, I. M., Oja, P. & Paronen, O. (1994) Physically active commuting to work–testing its potential for exercise promotion, *Medicine and Science in Sports and Exercise*, **26(7)**, 844–50.

Wandersman, A., Valois, R., Ochs, L., de la Cruz, D., Adkins, E. & Goodman, R. M. (1996) Toward a social ecology of community coalitions, *American Journal of Health Promotion*, **10**, 299–307.

9

Fitness Testing and Exercise Promotion – Issues and Recommendations

Lorraine Cale and Jo Harris

Physical fitness testing has been widely employed with young people for a number of years. Numerous fitness testing programmes, batteries, equipment, instruments and computer software have and still are being developed and promoted for use with young people, and the marketing and sale of such resources is clearly big business. As Chapter 3 revealed, fitness testing may be employed with young people in recreational programmes, public health surveys and assessments, and in clinical settings, though the most traditional and popular setting for fitness testing is in schools (ACSM, 2000). Evidence suggests that fitness testing is commonplace within the PE curriculum (Harris, 1995; ACSM, 2000), with most secondary schools including compulsory testing within their PE programmes (Ross et al., 1985; Harris,1995; Cale, 2000).

Yet, despite its popularity, controversy concerning fitness testing in young people has been on-going in recent decades and a number of issues have been raised and concerns expressed over the use of fitness tests with children (Fox & Biddle, 1986; Armstrong, 1987; 1989; ACSM, 1988; PEA, 1988; Seefeldt & Vogel, 1989; Safrit, 1990; Rowland, 1995; Harris & Cale, 1997; Cale & Harris, 1998; Harris, 2000). Issues concerning how much emphasis should be placed on physical fitness and physical fitness testing, the type, value and purpose of fitness testing, and the use, nature and structure of award systems have all been debated.

Clearly the relative merits and concerns of fitness testing need to be reviewed, and an informed discussion is required to consider the role of fitness testing in the promotion of exercise in young people. This chapter considers the key facts, issues, debates and recommendations concerning fitness testing as they relate to encouraging participation in a physically active lifestyle. Given the widespread practice of physical fitness testing in schools in particular, the focus of much of the discussion is on fitness testing within the PE curriculum. Nonetheless, the content presented is considered relevant and applicable to other settings.

Why the interest?

Physical fitness testing has perhaps assumed such popularity and interest for a variety of reasons. First, concerns over young people's physical fitness have attracted a good deal of attention in recent years. As Chapter 2 revealed, however, such concerns are ill-founded. Much media attention and 'hype' has been afforded to young people's fitness, with messages leading us to believe that all, or at least most, of today's youth are unfit, unhealthy, and far less fit than in previous decades. On this issue, Corbin (2002, p. 139) suggests that the media 'likes bad news' and that 'much talk about lack of fitness of our youth is hyperbole, designed to create a need for physical education in the eyes of the public'. Certainly, alarmed by such reports, PE teachers and others may feel compelled and even duty-bound to respond by focusing on and measuring young people's physical fitness. Indeed, the stimulus for a recent article by Cale & Harris (2002) was the confusion about fitness testing and questions from the profession as to whether national, standardized fitness tests should be introduced for all children as the 'way forward!' Such responses and suggestions are worrying and considered misguided on a number of counts (Cale & Harris, 2002), which will later become evident.

Secondly, in schools in England, it could be argued that the interest in fitness and testing is reinforced within and through the National Curriculum for Physical Education (NCPE). For example, it is noteworthy that the NCPE requirements refer to knowledge and understanding of 'fitness and health', and the terminology throughout the document is biased towards 'fitness' and 'training' (DfEE & QCA, 1999) rather than 'physical activity' and 'health'. Thirdly, the appeal of fitness testing to many teachers may be a consequence of the problems and concerns over monitoring and evaluation in PE (OFSTED, 1996). In the UK, guidance on 'what' and 'how' to assess in PE (see PEAUK, 2000), and more specifically within the area of health and fitness (Harris, 2000), has only recently been provided. It is perhaps not surprising therefore that, in the absence of alternative measures of attainment, fitness testing has become popular. It provides seemingly objective data on pupils' capabilities in a range of components of physical fitness. Finally, it is interesting to note that many health-related PE programmes (see Chapter 10) have focused on the development of children's physical fitness and, as a consequence, have typically been evaluated by performance measures on selected fitness tests (Harris & Cale, 1997).

Discussion point   Participating in physical fitness tests is among the most common memories many people hold – for better or worse – of their childhood PE experiences.

Did you encounter physical fitness testing at school? If so, what were your experiences and memories of fitness testing? Do you feel that these were typical of most pupils?

Have you had any other experiences of physical fitness testing (e.g. in different contexts) since leaving school? If so, what and how were these?

Overall, have your experiences of fitness testing been meaningful and positive, or meaningless and negative? Discuss your reasons.

Fitness tests – why? Why not?

As highlighted in Chapter 3, physical fitness testing in young people may be carried out in different settings for different reasons. Pate (1991) believes, however, that the most important reason for administering fitness tests is to facilitate learning in the cognitive and affective domains in terms of promoting knowledge and understanding of, and positive attitudes towards, exercise and fitness. Regrettably, however, he suggests that these aspects are also usually given the least attention.

Given that so many authors and organizations have expressed concerns over the use of fitness testing with young people (see earlier), this raises questions as to whether fitness tests do actually serve the purposes for which they are intended. First, whether tests provide a meaningful measure of young people's fitness is debatable. Monitoring young people's physical fitness is problematic, and it is generally accepted that fitness tests provide only a crude measure of an individual's physical fitness.

According to Fox & Biddle (1986), tests are plagued by severe limitations. The problems in monitoring young people's physical fitness are addressed in detail in Chapter 3. In summary, though, the appropriateness, validity and reliability of some fitness tests and fitness test batteries for use with children has been questioned (Safrit, 1990; Safrit & Looney, 1992; Rowland, 1995; Rice & Howell, 2000). The appropriateness of some tests is doubtful in that they have been developed for use with elite, adult populations (e.g. the Multistage Fitness Test) and are often applied to young people with little consideration of the differences between children's and adults' physiological and psychological responses to exercise (see Bar-Or, 1993). Indeed, the risks associated with using the Multistage Fitness Test with young people have been identified recently and safety advice has been given on how to reduce risks with the test (Eve & Williams, 2000). Similarly, the relevance and appropriateness of the mile run and other tests for children have also been queried (Hopple & Graham, 1995). Following reports from children that they did not enjoy taking the mile run, Hopple & Graham (1995, p. 416) remind us that children are not miniature adults, and claim that current tests 'which were designed by adults do not seem to mesh with children's perceptions of the world'. Interestingly, the distance run and the Multistage Fitness Test have been found to be the two most commonly employed fitness tests in schools in the UK (Harris, 1995). Such limitations and problems have led some to conclude that tests suitable for use in the school environment and which provide valid and objective measures of fitness are simply not available (PEA, 1988; Armstrong, 1989; Armstrong & Welsman, 1997).

In addition, the practice of applying norm and/or criterion-referenced standards in fitness testing is also known to have limitations. For example, norm tables do not indicate desired levels of physical fitness, provide any diagnostic feedback about whether fitness is adequate, and they imply that 'more is better' (Cureton, 1994). Equally, there is no evidence on the validity of criterion-referenced standards (Docherty & Bell, 1990; Safrit, 1990) and, because these standards represent desired minimum levels of fitness, it could be argued that they do not provide an incentive for young people to improve (Cureton, 1994) (see Chapter 3 for further details).

The limitations are perhaps better appreciated when one considers the many factors that influence fitness test performance. As Chapter 3 highlights, factors such as the environment/test conditions, lifestyle (exercise/nutrition), motivation, intellectual and mechanical skill at taking the test, test practice and, in particular, heredity or genetic potential and maturation all affect fitness performance and will be reflected in fitness test scores (Fox & Biddle, 1986; Docherty & Bell, 1990; Pangrazi, 2000). Indeed, the common definition of physical fitness which refers to 'a set of attributes that people have or achieve that relates to the ability to perform physical activity' (Caspersen, Powell and Christenson, 1985) suggests that physical fitness is partly a function of heredity (attributes that people have) as well as other factors (attributes that people achieve).

Despite the above, it is still often assumed that fitness in young people is primarily a reflection of the amount of activity performed, and that those who score highly on fitness tests are active and those who do not are inactive (Pangrazi, 2000). This assumption is inaccurate. The relationship between fitness and physical activity is low among children (Armstrong & Welsman, 1997) and a child's activity level cannot be judged from his or her fitness level (Corbin, 2002). According to Armstrong & Welsman (1997), the lack of relationship between physical activity and fitness probably lies in the low level of physical activity of most young people. Physical activity is an important variable in fitness development for adults, but for children and youth other factors are of equal or greater importance (Pangrazi, 2000). Clearly, in terms of promoting physical activity to young people, problems can arise if fitness test scores are linked to activity levels. On the one hand, an active child who scores poorly on a test may become disappointed, disillusioned, demotivated and 'turned off' activity because he/she feels it does not 'pay off' (Corbin, 2002). Equally, an inactive child who scores well may be delighted with the outcome, conclude that everything is all right when it is not, and consequently may not be motivated to change. Corbin (2002) illustrates the point, drawing parallels to dental health. He explains that children are taught that they must brush their teeth even if they do not have cavities – waiting for cavities to appear before brushing would be a mistake! Some children with good heredity, however, may have no cavities even if they do not brush their teeth, but they are still taught to brush anyway. In the same way, seemingly fit children who are inactive should learn the habit of activity when young, even if there is no evidence of low fitness.

A number of paradoxes relating to fitness testing have also been reported (Seefeldt & Vogel, 1989) which raise further questions over the relative merits of testing. For example, fitness tests purport to assess health-related physical fitness yet do not provide any clinical measures of health status (e.g. blood pressure, blood lipids), and they emphasize safe healthy practice yet some involve children performing tests which violate healthy behaviour. Further, Safrit (1990) explains that batteries claim to encourage the development of and maintenance of good fitness behaviours, but that the tests themselves do not always reflect this behaviour. For example, exercising to exhaustion as in the Multistage Fitness Test is not recommended practice, nor is executing as many sit-ups as possible in one minute. Indeed, Cale & Harris (2002) go so far as to suggest that these tests violate not only healthy behaviour but also common sense. Another paradox that relates to fitness tests is how they deprecate performance as a component of health-related fitness, yet in most test items performance is used as a basis for assessing fitness (Cale & Harris, 1998). Furthermore, the implications of fitness test per-formance for young people's health are not well established. There is only weak evidence that physical fitness is related to health in young people and no evidence that physical fitness during childhood and adolescence is related to adult health (Twisk, 2000) (see Chapter 2). The same, however, is also true of physical activity and more research is clearly needed. Yet it is proposed that until more evidence is available supporting the relationship between childhood fitness characteristics and childhood and adult health, and for reasons which will now be explained, more attention should be given to young people's physical activity levels. The issue of fitness versus activity is considered later and discussed in more detail in Chapter 2.

A further and important consideration is how test procedures might affect the social, emotional and attitudinal values of young people towards activity (Seefeldt & Vogel, 1989; Cale & Harris, 2002). Concern has been expressed that fitness testing may be counterproductive to the promotion of active lifestyles in young people (Docherty & Bell, 1990; Corbin, Pangrazi & Welk, 1995; Rowland, 1995). According to Rowland (1995), fitness tests are anti-ethical to the goal of promoting physical activity in children in so far as they can be demeaning, embarrassing and uncomfortable for children (often those about whom there is most concern), and may reinforce the notion that exercise is competitive and unpleasant. Docherty & Bell (1990) claim that fitness tests are frequently misused, which can have negative consequences on physical activity participation. Similarly, Corbin, Pangrazi & Welk (1995) warn that testing which is done improperly may turn many youngsters 'off' rather than 'on' to activity and should therefore be discontinued. Tests may also communicate a false message to young people, namely that com-petition and excellence are necessary for health and fitness, which may further confound the goal of promoting physical activity.

On the issue of excellence, it is acknowledged that fitness testing might be used to identify youngsters with athletic potential (Pate, 1994) and/or help the elite prepare for sports participation (Corbin, Pangrazi & Welk, 1995). Pate (1994), however, suggests that whilst fitness test results can provide some information that is useful in guiding youngsters into appropriate athletics activities, the benefits in this area are probably quite limited. This is because contemporary fitness testing procedures do not usually focus on those fitness components, such as speed, anaerobic power and agility, that are important in many of the most popular athletic activities. Also, performance in most athletic activities depends on a complex mix of factors including specific motor skill performance, motivation and experience, as well as fitness. Corbin, Pangrazi & Welk (1995) believe that tests for these purposes are not for all youth and that they should be conducted after school or in practice sessions.

Advocates of physical fitness testing in schools argue that testing motivates young people to maintain or enhance their physical fitness or physical activity levels, increases knowledge and promotes physical activity via fostering positive attitudes (see Chapter 3). However, whilst a good deal of research has been conducted on measurement issues and the reliability and validity of fitness tests in recent years, surprisingly little attention has been paid to the motivational effects of fitness testing on young people or young people's perspectives of, or knowledge and/or attitudes towards, tests (Fox & Biddle, 1988; Jackson, 2000). Given the prevalence of fitness testing among young people, and from a physical activity promotion perspective, the impact of tests, their educational value and the way in they are perceived by young people would seem to be crucial in determining the appropriateness or otherwise of their use in schools. The need for research of this nature was recognized by Pate in 1991 who suggested: 'It would be desirable to know how children respond to participation in these (physical fitness) tests. Are tests viewed as fun? Do tests have differential effects on different types of children?' (Pate, 1991, p. 233).

Whitehead & Corbin (1991) investigated the effect of fitness testing on motivation in youth and found that intrinsic motivation increased as a result of positive feedback after the test but decreased following negative feedback. These variations were also mediated by perceived competence. Goudas, Biddle & Fox (1994) found that different children have different motivational reactions to fitness testing, depending on their achievement goal orientation, performance and perceived success. They concluded that the effects of fitness testing are complex and that motivational enhancement following testing cannot be taken for granted. Likewise, the PEA has also noted that there is no hard evidence that fitness tests motivate individuals and suggest that in parallel areas of education there is supportive evidence that tests only motivate those who do well (PEA, 1988).

Concerning knowledge and attitudes, Hopple & Graham (1995) investigated what children 'thought, felt and knew about' the mile run test. They revealed that children generally showed little or no under-standing of why they were being asked to complete the test and many disliked taking it, viewing it as a painful, negative experience to be either actively or passively 'dodged'. Adams (1996), meanwhile, investigated the effects of student attitudes toward PE and exercise on the mile run test and concluded that a positive attitude towards PE was related to children's performance on the mile run. Lastly, a study of adolescents' attitudes toward school PE revealed that young people viewed fitness testing unfavourably and as a major contributor to negative attitudes towards PE (Luke & Sinclair, 1991). Interestingly, programmes designed to increase knowledge and appreciation of the role and value of exercise on physical fitness and health have been reported to be virtually non-existent in schools in the US (ACSM, 1988).

There is also concern that the administration of fitness tests could lead to more attention being given to product-related issues such as 'fit-ness' and 'performance' within a PE programme than to process-oriented issues such as 'health' and 'physical activity' behaviour (Harris & Cale, 1997; Cale & Harris, 2002). From a public health and physical activity promotion perspective, it is argued that the goal should be to influence the 'process', i.e. physical activity, rather than the 'product' of fitness for a number of reasons (Rowland, 1995; Pangrazi, 2000; Cale & Harris, 2002; Corbin, 2002). Corbin (2002) argues that the idea that physical fitness is a paramount goal for children is a misconception and reminds us that focusing too much on fitness can have as many negative consequences as positive ones. It is also claimed that the focus on raising fitness levels which was common practice for many years, has been unsuccessful (Pangrazi, 2000). In contrast, raised physical activity is an outcome that can be accomplished by all children regardless of ability (or disability) or personal interests, and will further benefit those young people who need it most (Pangrazi, 2000). Because physical activity monitoring is free from genetic and maturational influences, it effectively 'levels the playing field', allowing all to succeed. Similarly, Rowland (1995) suggests that a shift in promoting physical activity is more likely to be acceptable to the general public, particularly to those who are sedentary or have low fitness levels. Indeed, he views the routine field testing of children as 'archaic and inconsistent with our current understanding of the exercise-health connection' (p. 125) and claims that a shift from a fitness to a physical activity promotion model would serve as the best argument for abandoning the practice.

Thus, we need to help young people understand the importance of being active, to realise that their fitness levels may not be a good indicator of their physical activity participation, and to appreciate the limitations of testing and the range of factors that account for an individual's fitness. Indeed, it is encouraging to note that some of the more recent fitness test batteries now recognize the importance of physical activity as well as fitness. The goals of FITNESSGRAM, for example, are to promote enjoyable regular physical activity and to provide comprehensive physical fitness *and activity* assessments and reporting programmes for children and youth (Cooper Institute for Aerobics Research, 1999). The programme furthermore seeks to develop affective, cognitive and behavioural components related to participation in regular physical activity.

To date, research findings also highlight the need to focus attention on influencing young people's physical activity behaviour rather than their physical fitness. Evidence suggests that a sizeable proportion of young people are inactive and lead sedentary lifestyles. By comparison, however, there is no evidence that low levels of aerobic fitness are common amongst young people or that their fitness has declined over the past 50 years (see Chapter 2).

That said, whilst a shift in emphasis towards physical activity has been called for, researchers have also warned that physical fitness should not be abandoned. Boreham & Riddoch (2001) claim that the question of whether physical activity or fitness is most strongly related to health status remains unresolved, and report that the evidence that fitness is related to young people's health itself, without being mediated by physical activity, is becoming increasingly persuasive. Given the strong and consistent relationships between activity or fitness and health in adults, they conclude that it is probable that ensuring adequate activity *and fitness* in children will be of ultimate benefit (see Chapter 2).

Finally, there are concerns with the way in which fitness tests are implemented and conducted within the curriculum. According to Pate (1989), too often tests have been an almost irrelevant adjunct to the curriculum. Also, they often dominate programmes and in some cases constitute the entire fitness education programme. The amount of curriculum time spent on fitness testing without necessarily positively influencing young people's activity levels or their attitudes towards physical activity has been criticized (Harris & Cale, 1997; Cale & Harris, 2002). For the reasons already outlined, fitness tests are not necessarily beneficial for the promotion of exercise and physical activity, which suggests that PE time could sometimes be used more wisely. The time spent on performing and scoring fitness tests may detract from promoting the process of being active (Harris, 2000) and may be at the expense of time spent on more useful exercise-promoting activities, and of developing knowledge and understanding about physical fitness and what physical fitness tests measure. Administering fitness tests simply to acquire data for records, without attention to their educational role, is not advised (Harris, 2000). Indeed, studies of teachers' perspectives of fitness testing have identified time as a major barrier to fitness testing in the curriculum (Veal, 1988; Jackson, 2000).

In terms of conducting fitness tests, Corbin, Pangrazi & Welk (1995, p. 348) ask, 'is it the testing itself that is 'bad' or the way in which it is done?' Clearly, if tests are to achieve cognitive, affective and behavioural objectives, then they need to be implemented and conducted thoughtfully, sensitively and in accordance with good pedagogical practice. The following 'recommendations' section addresses this issue (see Table 9.1).

Finally, the way in which fitness test results are used is important. Fitness test scores may be put to a number of uses, some of which may be considered inappropriate and undesirable. For example, test scores have been used to grade pupils as a primary indicator of achievement in PE, to evaluate teacher competence, or as a measure of the success of an institution or programme (Corbin, Pangrazi & Welk, 1995; Corbin 2002). Employing fitness tests for such purposes, however, has been challenged. Corbin (2002) is highly critical of schools that use fitness test scores for such purposes. He suggests such schools obviously and mistakenly subscribe to the idea that fitness is the paramount goal of PE, and warns that this could have the following potential negative consequences:

- loss of interest in PE and physical activity
- teaching to the test

- student and teacher cheating on fitness tests
- undermining the confidence of students who find that, even with effort, they cannot achieve the fitness goals necessary to get good grades or to meet teacher expectations. (Corbin, 2002, pp. 134–5)

Some of these consequences may seem extreme, but are indeed legitimate if test scores are, as we are led to believe, commonly used for such purposes (Corbin, Pangrazi & Welk, 1995; Corbin 2002). Armstrong & Welsman (1997, p. 257) advise, 'teachers must ask themselves why they are testing young people's fitness, and if the answer is for classification purposes, then we suggest that they would be better employed seriously addressing the problem of young people's sedentary lifestyles'. In our view, and taking into account the limitations of fitness testing and the many factors which influence test scores, it seems ridiculous to suggest that the success or otherwise of programmes and/or pupils in PE should be determined by young people's fitness levels, or that teachers should in some way be held accountable for the fitness levels of their pupils.

Case study (to be conducted in a group of 4–6)
You are all members of a PE department and are currently reviewing your PE curriculum. Based on your knowledge of fitness testing, the department must decide whether to include fitness testing within the PE curriculum or not. What decision do you make and why?

Recommendations

Given the preceding analysis, it is perhaps not surprising that fitness testing with young people has come under such scrutiny in recent years. Fitness testing can be a fruitless and/or counterproductive activity. Without careful consideration of the issues, limitations and factors influencing fitness tests, and the way in which tests are administered, fitness testing can be unpleasant, embarrassing and meaningless for many young people, and scores can be inaccurate, misleading, unfair and demotivating. According to Pate (1994), concerns about the impact of fitness testing on young people's attitudes towards physical activity and fitness in particular have forced a re-examination of the role of fitness tests in PE in recent years. Others are of the view that fitness testing might survive only if it can be shown that it promotes the right philosophy (Corbin, Pangrazi & Welk, 1995).

However, there is no reason why fitness testing cannot promote the right philosophy. We should not lose sight of the fact that, if appropriately employed, and provided all relevant factors are taken into account, fitness testing can play a valuable role in the promotion of physical activity and in educating young people about physical activity and fitness. In a position statement, the Fitness and Health Advisory Committee of the PEA concluded that

Fitness testing and monitoring can be valuable components of a health-related fitness programme if they are used:

i)   encourage positive attitudes towards health-related fitness;
ii) increase understanding of the principles underlying health-related fitness; and
iii) promote a lifetime commitment to health-related fitness. (PEA, 1988, p. 194)

To achieve the above, it would seem that clear guidance on the use of fitness testing in young people is needed. Surprisingly, though, despite its popularity over a number of years, there is little scientific evidence to guide us in deciding how best to incorporate fitness testing into PE (Pate, 1994). As already noted, most of the research in this area has addressed issues of measurement, validity and reliability. Little attention has been paid to understanding how young people respond to fitness tests or how tests can best be used to attain important educational and physical activity promotion objectives. Recommendations concerning the implementation of fitness testing with young people have been made by a number of researchers and professional organizations (e.g. ACSM, 1988; Harris & Elbourn, 1994; Pate, 1994; Pate & Hohn, 1994; Corbin, Pangrazi & Welk, 1995; AAHPERD (American Alliance for Health, Physical Education, Recreation and Dance), 1999a; 1999b; 1999c; Harris, 2000), but these have been based more on common sense that on scientific evidence. A summary and interpretation of the key recommendations and messages found in the literature is presented in Table 9.1. In addition, teachers may need specific support and training in the implementation of physical fitness testing within the curriculum and, in particular, in how to use tests and test results to achieve cognitive, affective and behavioural objectives with young people.

Table 9.1 Fitness testing – recommendations

General

Fitness testing should not dominate a PE programme, neither should it be an adjunct to it. It should be fully and appropriately integrated into the curriculum.

Fitness testing should be used to encourage and help young people acquire and maintain fitness levels that are appropriate for their personal needs. It should be recognized that the majority of youngsters are sufficiently 'fit' and that 'high level' fitness is not necessary for all young people.

Content

Fitness testing should focus on monitoring the health-related components of fitness (i.e. cardiovascular fitness, flexibility, muscular strength and endurance, and possibly body composition (if dealt with sensitively)).

Tests batteries should be developmentally appropriate and include developmentally appropriate exercises (e.g. different versions of exercises). Tests designed for adults should be avoided, or modified and sub-maximal tests selected.

It should not be assumed that fitness testing will increase pupils' activity levels. The development and maintenance of lifelong activity habits should be addressed and activity promotion measures included (e.g. monitoring activity; raising awareness and providing access to activity opportunities; goal setting, self monitoring and self-evaluation) alongside testing.

Organization/Delivery

Testing should be child-centred and accessible for all young people. Personal improvement over time should be the focus, not comparisons with others.

Fitness testing should be a positive and meaningful experience presented in an individualized manner that provides young people with personalized baseline scores and feedback from which to improve their activity and fitness levels. Testing should never be administered at the expense of an individual's self-concept or confidence. The public nature of testing should be minimized and prior practice given on tests to make young people feel comfortable and at ease and to allow them to perform their best. If body composition is measured, this should be done so sensitively and as privately as possible. Compulsory use of exhausting maximal tests should be avoided. It may be appropriate to incorporate fitness testing as a choice activity.

Table 9.1 (Continued)

Fitness testing should promote learning, and health-related learning concepts should be delivered during the fitness testing process (e.g. explaining the relevance of each component and ensuring that young people understand how to improve each component).

Fitness testing should adhere to and be consistent with good practice (e.g. it should incorporate a warm-up and cool-down, safe exercise practices, familiarization with the testing procedures, and be conducted in a safe environment – well ventilated, adequate space, with appropriate equipment, etc.).

Fitness testing should be made as much fun, and as varied and relevant as possible, and move beyond 'traditional' administration methods. For example, student choices, testing options, home tasks, self and partner/peer (vs. whole-group) assessments, encouragement of self-responsibility and goal setting, and the use of fun equipment may hold merit and be more developmentally appropriate and relevant ways of testing young people's fitness.

Feedback/Evaluation

Fitness test results should be communicated and used with young people in a meaningful way that promotes affective and cognitive learning about maintaining and/or improving personal fitness. Fitness test scores should be interpreted and explained carefully, with recognition of their limitations.

If standards are used in interpreting scores, they should be explained, and criterion-referenced rather than normative standards should be employed. (Criterion-referenced standards are attainable by the vast majority of young people and reinforce the fitness–health link and the notion that one can be fit without being an elite athlete).

Whilst all young people should be provided with feedback, it is particularly important that youngsters identified as very low fit are provided with appropriate and sensitive remedial support, encouragement and progress monitoring. This might involve suggestions for activities/exercises they can undertake in their leisure time at home or in the local community, communication with parents or, in extreme circumstances, referral to their GP.

Test re-test procedures (e.g. administering a test at the beginning and again at the end of a unit of work, school year) should be implemented with caution and only if the intervening programme/unit was designed to produce change and promote 'fitness'. Even then, programmes/units are often too short (6–8 weeks) to expect any real changes and testing could have a demotivating effect. The practice can also be time-consuming and detract from learning time.

The use of external rewards or award schemes can be a useful and legitimate tool for motivating young people but should be used sparingly. They should not be used to bribe children or to reward performance. If employed, they should reward and encourage activity objectives (not fitness performance) and should be attainable by all young people.

Home influences on young people's activity and fitness levels should be recognized in feedback/evaluation and parents/guardians should be encouraged to show interest in their children's physical activity and physical fitness and to be positive role models.

Table 9.2 Alternative ways of monitoring achievement in 'health and fitness'

Assessment via:	Examples
Pupils' responses to focused questions and practical tasks	Why is it important to stretch muscles after you have worked them? Perform an exercise to strengthen your stomach Demonstrate 3 exercises that will raise your heart rate
Teacher observation of pupils' performance in practical tasks	Do the pupils apply their understanding? Do the pupils perform the exercises/activities with correct technique?
Pupils taking more responsibility for their actions within and outside lessons	Can the pupils work independently in lessons and make appropriate decisions? Are the pupils participating in activity out of school?
Pupils' attendance, participation and commitment in PE lessons and to extra-curricular activities	The number of PE lessons missed or not participated in The degree of interest shown and effort put into lessons
Pupils' participation in physical activity outside of school	Membership or involvement in clubs, activities and events

Source: Cale & Harris (2002) Reproduced with permission.

Table 9.3 Health and fitness assessment tasks

	Assessment Tasks		
Warming up and cooling down	**Activity opportunities**	**Keeping an activity diary**	**Planning and evaluating an exercise programme**
Level Description – 5 'Pupils warm up and cool down in ways that suit the activity'.	**Level description – 6 'Pupils describe how they might get involved in other types of activities and exercise'.**	**Level Description – 7 'Pupils explain the principles of practice and training, and apply them effectively'.**	**Level Description – 8 'Pupils use their knowledge of health and fitness to plan and evaluate their own exercise and activity programme'.**
1) Working by yourself or with one other person, plan a 10 minute warm-up and a 5 minute cool-down for either: sprinting; soccer; tennis; or an energetic dance performance.	1) How can you find out about the activity opportunities available to you in your local area (e.g. from who and from where)? Make a list of the individuals you could contact and the sources you could go to.	1) Keep an activity diary for 2–3 weeks. Record the type and amount of activity you do each day. Also, make a note of how hard the activity was (light, moderate or difficult).	1) What factors do you need to consider when planning your exercise programme? How long should your exercise programme be? Why do you think this is? What should it include and why?

The warm-up/cool-down should include:
- actions which relate to the activity you are warming up for/ cooling down from
- activities that gradually increase your heart rate and breathing and warm your body or which gradually decrease your heart rate and breathing and cool your body
- a few mobility exercises in the warm-up for joints that you will be using in the activity
- 2 or 3 stretches for muscles which are going to be worked hard or which have been worked hard during the activity.

2) What information about the activity do you need to know/find out? Make a list of the questions you would need to ask.
3) Research an activity of your choice. Think of an activity you would like to try and, using the library, the internet or any other source of information, try to find out some or all of the following information about the activity:
- What does the activity involve?
- What are the general rules or procedures that must be followed?
- How many people do you need to take part?
- What equipment and clothing does the activity require?

2) At the end of the 2–3 weeks, look back over your physical activity and explain how successful you feel you have been in adhering to the following important principles of training:
- Overload
- Progression
- Specificity
- Balance, moderation and variety
- Maintenance
Why do you think these principles are important?

2) Write week one of your exercise programme. Then write your programme for the next few weeks.
3) Evaluating your exercise programme:
Why do you think it is important to evaluate your exercise programme?
What changes in yourself, if any, have you noticed from your exercise programme?
Record any changes you have noticed in your:
- activity patterns (more active; engage in more variety of activities)
- physical fitness (feel fitter; muscles feel and look more toned; joints are looser and more agile)

Table 9.3 (Continued)

Assessment Tasks

Warming up and Cooling down	Activity Opportunities	Keeping an activity diary	Planning and evaluating an exercise programme
Level Description – 5 'Pupils warm up and cool down in ways that suit the activity.'	**Level description – 6 'Pupils describe how they might get involved in other types of activities and exercise.'**	**Level Description – 7 'Pupils explain the principles of practice and training, and apply them effectively.'**	**Level Description – 8 'Pupils use their knowledge of health and fitness to plan and evaluate their own exercise and activity programme.'**
2) Afterwards, for either the warm-up or cool-down, explain to another person/pair: which actions were related to the activity you were warming up for/cooling down from?	– Where, when and how can you get involved? 4) Contribute to a class activity directory of the activities available in your local area. What information would you need to record in the directory? How would you organise and present the information? Design a sample page of the activity directory.		– general health (feel better; more energy; lost some body fat) – mental health (feel happier; in a better mood; more confident) If you have not noticed many changes, why do you think this is? What has influenced your exercise programme?

- how the activities gradually increased your heart rate and breathing/decreased your heart rate and breathing?
- which stretches were relevant to the activity
- which exercises in the warm-up/cool-down were for the joints used in the activity?
- why you consider the warm-up/cool-down was effective and relevant

What factors have helped you with your exercise programme? What constraints have hindered you? Can you think of ways round these?

Source: Cale & Harris (2002) Reproduced with permission.

Discussion point   Refer to the recommendations for fitness testing in Table 9.1. Within a group situation (e.g. a PE class or a training session within a sports club), what measures could be taken to ensure that fitness testing is: (1) accessible and (2) a positive, meaningful and relevant experience for the following young people:

1   an overweight child?
2   a gifted and talented athlete?
3   a late-maturing child who is particularly small for his/her age?
4   a child in a wheelchair?
5   a timid child with little self-confidence or self-esteem?

Alternatives to fitness testing

Fitness testing in schools is acceptable, provided it is appropriately conducted, but it is certainly not essential, and formal testing of primary-aged schoolchildren is not recommended (Harris, 2000). Given this, and the many issues surrounding fitness testing in young people, some teachers may decide to abandon tests in favour of alternative methods of monitoring young people. However, even if teachers retain fitness testing, this should ideally be complemented via other methods of assessment.

As recommended, if young people are to be encouraged to focus not only on the 'product' of fitness but also on the 'process' of activity, then this should be reflected in the assessment methods that are employed. According to Harris (2000), achievement in health and fitness relates to improvements in knowledge and understanding, competence and motor skills, behavioural skills, and attitudes and confidence, which could be monitored in a variety of ways. A number of alternative means by which young people's progress and achievement in this area can be measured have been proposed, with specific examples provided (e.g. see AAHPERD, 1999a; 1999b; 1999c; Cale & Harris, 2002). A summary of the methods and example health and fitness assessment tasks proposed by Cale & Harris (2002) are shown in Tables 9.2 and 9.3. Table 9.3 identifies tasks intended for secondary-aged pupils (Key Stages 3 and 4) and the NCPE (National Curriculum for Physical Education) level descriptors to which they relate. As can be seen, the methods and tasks include assessment of the behavioural, cognitive and affective as well as physical domains. According to preference, these methods could be used as a substitute for, or alongside, physical fitness testing within the curriculum.

References

AAHPERD (American Alliance for Health, Physical Education, Recreation and Dance) (1999a) *Physical Education for Lifelong Fitness. The Physical Best Teachers' Guide*. Champaign, IL: Human Kinetics.

AAHPERD (American Alliance for Health, Physical Education, Recreation and Dance) (1999b) *Physical Best Activity Guide. Secondary Level*. Champaign, IL: Human Kinetics.

AAHPERD (American Alliance for Health, Physical Education, Recreation and Dance) (1999c) *Physical Best Activity Guide. Elementary Level*. Champaign, IL: Human Kinetics.

ACSM (American College of Sports Medicine) (1988) Opinion statement on physical fitness in children and youth, *Medicine and Science in Sport and Exercise*, **20(4)**, 422–3.

ACSM (American College of Sports Medicine) (2000) Exercise testing and prescription for children, the elderly, and pregnant women. In *ACSM's Guidelines for Exercise Testing and Prescription*, 6th edn. Philadelphia, PA: Lippincott Williams & Wilkins, 217–34.

Adams, T. M. (1996) An investigation of the effects of student attitudes towards physical education and exercise on selected health related fitness test parameters (abstract), *Research Quarterly for Exercise and Sport Supplement*, **March**, A–39.

Armstrong, N. (1987) A critique of fitness testing. In Biddle, S. (ed.), *Foundations of Health Related Fitness in Physical Education*. London: Ling Publishing House, 19–27.

Armstrong, N. (1989) Is fitness testing either valid or useful? *British Journal of Physical Education*, **20**, 66–7.

Armstrong, N. & Welsman, J. (1997) *Young People and Physical Activity*. Oxford: Oxford University Press.

Bar-Or, O. (1993) Importance of differences between children and adults for exercise testing and exercise prescription. In Skinner, J. S. (ed.), *Exercise Testing and Prescription for Special Cases*, 2nd edn. Philadelphia, PA, Lea & Febiger, 57–74.

Boreham, C. & Riddoch, C. (2001) The physical activity, fitness and health of children, *Journal of Sports Science*, **19**, 915–29.

Cale, L. (2000) Physical activity promotion in secondary schools, *European Physical Education Review*, **6(1)**, 71–90.

Cale, L. & Harris, J. (1998) The benefits of health-related physical education and recommendations for implementation, *The Bulletin of Physical Education*, **34(1)**, 27–41.

Cale, L. & Harris, J. (2002) National fitness testing for children – issues, concerns and alternatives, *The British Journal of Teaching Physical Education*, **33(1)**, 32–4.

Caspersen, C. J., Powell, K. E. & Christenson, G. M. (1985) Physical activity, exercise and physical fitness: definitions and distinctions for health-related research, *Public Health Reports*, **100**, 126–30.

Cooper Institute for Aerobics Research (1999) *FITNESSGRAM. Test Administration Manual*, 2nd edn. Champaign, IL: Human Kinetics.

Corbin, C. B. (2002) Physical activity for everyone: what every physical educator should know about promoting lifelong physical activity, *Journal of Teaching in Physical Education*, **21**, 128–44.

Corbin, C. B., Pangrazi, R. P. & Welk, G. J. (1995) A response to 'The horse is dead; let's dismount', *Pediatric Exercise Science*, **7**, 347–51.

Cureton, K. J. (1994) Physical fitness and activity standards for youth. In Pate, R. R. & Hohn, R. C. (eds), *Health and Fitness Through Physical Education*. Champaign, IL: Human Kinetics, 129–36.

DfEE & QCA (Department for Education and Employment & Qualifications and Curriculum Authority) (1999) *Physical Education. The National Curriculum for England*. London: HMSO.

Docherty, D. & Bell, R. (1990) Fitness testing: counterproductive to a healthy lifestyle? *CAHPER Journal*, **56(5)**, 4–8.

Eve, N. & Williams, D. (2000) Multistage fitness test in secondary schools – advice on safety, *Bulletin of Physical Education*, **36(2)**, 110–14.

Fox, K. & Biddle, S. (1986) Health related fitness testing in schools: introduction and problems of interpretation, *The Bulletin of Physical Education*, **22**, 54–64.

Fox, K. R. & Biddle, S. J. H. (1988) The use of fitness tests: educational and psychological considerations, *Journal of Physical Education Recreation and Dance*, **59(2)**, 47–53.

Goudas, M., Biddle, S. & Fox, K. (1994) Achievement goal orientations and intrinsic motivation in physical fitness testing with children, *Pediatric Exercise Science*, **6**, 159–67.

Harris, J. (1995) Physical education – a picture of health?, *The British Journal of Physical Education*, **26(4)**, 25–32.

Harris, J. (2000) *Health-Related Exercise in the National Curriculum. Key Stages 1 to 4*. Leeds: Human Kinetics.

Harris, J. & Cale, L. (1997) How healthy is school PE? A review of the effectiveness of health-related physical education programmes in schools, *Health Education Journal*, **56**, 84–104.

Harris, J. & Elbourn, J. (1994) Measure for measure. Does activity and fitness monitoring have a place within physical education? *Sports Teacher*, **Autumn**, 11–15.

Hopple, C. & Graham, G. (1995) What children think, feel and know about physical fitness testing, *Journal of Teaching in Physical Education*, **14(4)**, 408–17.

Jackson, J. A. (2000) Fitness testing: student and teacher perspectives, *AAHPERD Journal of Health, Physical Education, Recreation and Dance*, **38(3)**, 29–31.

Luke, M. D. & Sinclair, G. D. (1991) Gender differences in adolescents' attitudes toward school physical education, *Journal of Teaching in Physical Education*, **11**, 31–46.

Office for Standards in Education (OFSTED) (1996) *Subjects and Standards. Issues for School Development Arising from OFSTED Inspection Findings 1994/95. Key Stages 3 and 4 and Post 16*. London: HMSO.

Pangrazi, R. P. (2000) Promoting physical activity for youth, *The ACHPER Healthy Lifestyles Journal*, **47(2)**, 18–21.

Pate, R. (1991) Health-related measures of children's physical fitness, *Journal of School Health*, **61**, 231–3.

Pate, R. R. (1989) The case for large-scale physical fitness testing in American youth, *Pediatric Exercise Science*, **1**, 290–4.

Pate, R. R. (1994) Fitness testing: current approaches and purposes in physical education. In Pate, R. R. & Hohn, R. C. (eds), *Health and Fitness through Physical Education*. Champaign, IL: Human Kinetics, 119–27.

Pate, R. R. & Hohn, R. C. (1994) Health-related physical education – a direction for the 21st century. In Pate, R. R. & Hohn, R. C. (eds), *Health and Fitness through Physical Education*. Champaign, IL: Human Kinetics, 215–17.

PEA (Physical Education Association) (1988) Health related fitness testing and monitoring in schools. A position statement on behalf of the PEA by its fitness and health advisory committee, *British Journal of Physical Education*, **19(4/5)**, 194–5.

PEAUK (Physical Education Association of the United Kingdom) (2000) *Guidance Materials for National Curriculum 2000. Assessment, Recording and Reporting at Key Stages 1 to 4*. Reading: PEAUK.

Rice, M. H. & Howell, C. C. (2000) Measurement of physical activity, exercise and physical fitness in children: issues and concerns, *Journal of Pediatric Nursing*, **15(3)**, 148–56.

Ross, J. G., Dotson, C. O., Gilbert, G. G. & Katz, S. J. (1985) What are kids doing in school physical education? *Journal of Physical Education, Recreation and Dance*, **56**, 73–6.

Rowland, T. W. (1995) The horse is dead; let's dismount, *Pediatric Exercise Science*, **7**, 117–20.

Safrit, M. (1990) The validity and reliability of fitness tests for children: a review, *Pediatric Exercise Science*, **2**, 9–28.

Safrit, M. J. & Looney, M. A. (1992) Should the punishment fit the crime? A measurement dilemma, *Research Quarterly for Exercise and Sport*, **62**, 24–127.

Seefeldt, V. & Vogel, P. (1989) Physical fitness testing of children: a 30-year history of misguided efforts, *Pediatric Exercise Science*, **1**, 295–302.

Twisk, J. W. R. (2000) Physical activity, physical fitness and cardiovascular health. In Armstrong, N. & Van Mechelen, W. (eds), *Paediatric Exercise Science and Medicine*. Oxford: Oxford University Press, 253–63.

Veal, M. L. (1988) Pupil assessment perceptions and practices of secondary teachers, *Journal of Teaching in Physical Education*, **7**, 327–42.

Whitehead, J. R. & Corbin, C. B. (1991) Youth fitness testing: the effect of percentile-based evaluative feedback on intrinsic motivation, *Research Quarterly for Exercise and Sport*, **62**, 225–31.

10

Physical Activity Promotion Interventions, Initiatives, Resources and Contacts

Lorraine Cale and Jo Harris

The first part of this chapter considers school- and community-based interventions that have been designed to increase young people's physical activity participation. The outcomes of formally evaluated physical activity interventions are reviewed and the trends, characteristics and a number of issues concerning such interventions are highlighted. To conclude, the chapter turns attention to a range of UK initiatives, resources and contact organizations which can support the promotion of physical activity among young people.

Physical activity interventions

School-based interventions

As highlighted in Chapter 7, the promotion of physical activity within schools and the PE curriculum has attracted growing interest in recent years. According to Stone and colleagues (1998), school-based physical activity interventions have an inherent advantage over interventions in other settings because programmes can become institutionalized into the regular school curriculum, staff development and other infrastructures. It is perhaps not surprising, therefore, that they are the most common form of intervention for young people. A number of studies of varying degrees of rigour have been conducted to evaluate the effectiveness of school-based interventions over the past decade and, more recently, reviews have been published which have considered their effectiveness (see Harris & Cale, 1997; Almond & Harris, 1998; Stone et al., 1998; Kahn et al., 2002).

Harris & Cale (1997) and Almond & Harris (1998) conducted a review of studies of formally evaluated primary and secondary school health-related PE (HRPE) programmes, predominately from the US, the UK, Canada and Australia. Stone et al. (1998) conducted a review and synthesis of physical activity interventions in youth, employing stricter study-inclusion criteria whereby only studies that had used a quantitative assessment of physical activity and a comparison or control group were included. A total of 14 completed school-based studies met these criteria, 11 of which were conducted in the US. A further five studies were reported to be in progress.

More recently, Kahn et al. (2002) undertook a systematic review of the effectiveness of various approaches to increasing physical activity. Only studies considered to be of at least fair design or execution were included. Ten studies were reviewed which evaluated the effectiveness of classroom-based health education programmes, three which evaluated classroom-based programmes that focused on reducing TV viewing and video-game playing, and thirteen which evaluated the effectiveness of modified PE programmes.

Intervention findings

Studies which have evaluated the effectiveness of classroom-based health education programmes have shown variable effects on physical activity. Some studies revealed increases in physical activity (e.g. the Australia School Study (Homel et al., 1981); the Southwest Cardiovascular (CV) Curriculum Project (Davis et al., 1995)), and others revealed decreases (e.g. the Slice of Life Project (Perry et al., 1987)). A few studies showed improvements in knowledge, attitude and self-efficacy about exercise (e.g. the Slice of Life Project; the Southwest CV Curriculum Project).

The few classroom-based programmes that focused on reducing TV viewing and video-game playing (Gortmaker et al., 1999a; 1999b; Robinson, 1999) found a consistent and sizeable decrease in TV viewing and video-game playing and, in one study, time spent in other sedentary behaviours also decreased (Robinson, 1999). However, reductions in TV viewing and video-game playing did not consistently correspond with increases in physical activity.

Consistent increases in time spent in physical activity at school were observed in the studies which had implemented modified PE programmes (Kahn et al., 2002). Increases in the amount or percentage of time spent in moderate-to-vigorous physical activity (MVPA) in PE classes were found in a number of studies (e.g. Dwyer et al., 1983; Go for Health (Parcel et al., 1989; Simons-Morton et al., 1991); the Child and Adolescent Trial for Cardiovascular Health (CATCH) (Luepker et al., 1996; McKenzie et al., 1996); the Nebraska School Study (Donnelly et al., 1996); Sports, Play and Active Recreation for Kids (SPARK) (McKenzie et al., 1997; Sallis et al., 1997)). Indeed, the net increase in the amount of PE class time spent in MVPA was reported to be 50.3 per cent (Kahn et al., 2002). Increases in energy expenditure were also reported in a few studies (e.g. CATCH; SPARK).

Few positive findings, however, were reported for out-of-school physical activity. Some studies reported significant increases in out-of-school activity (e.g. CATCH; the Oslo Youth Study (Tell & Vellar, 1987); the Australia School Study; the Stanford Adolescent Heart Health Study (Killen et al., 1988)), but others did not (e.g. Go for Health; SPARK). Indeed, whilst the Nebraska School Study reported a significant increase in physical activity during school PE, less out-of-school activity was reported for the intervention group.

Studies also showed increases in measures of physical fitness (e.g. Hopper et al., 1992; Shephard & Lavallee, 1993; 1994; the Oslo Youth Study; the Path Program (Fardy, White & Haltiwanger-Schmitz, 1996); SPARK; Pieron et al., 1996; Manios et al., 1999). The majority of studies also examined weight change but the results were inconsistent. Finally, these interventions were also associated with increased knowledge (e.g. Go for Health; the Oslo Youth Study; Hopper et al., 1992; the Cardiovascular Health in Children Study (CHIC) (Harrell et al., 1996); the Path Program; the Stanford Adolescent Heart Health Programme), improved attitudes (e.g. Go for Health; Pieron et al., 1996) and self-efficacy (CATCH; Go for Health).

On the basis of these findings, it would seem that school-based PE programmes can achieve a range of positive outcomes (Harris & Cale, 1997; Almond & Harris, 1998). Meaningful improvements in activity and fitness levels, and in knowledge and attitudes, have been reported following school-based studies. Kahn and colleagues (2002) concluded from their review that there is strong evidence that school-based PE is effective in increasing levels of physical activity and improving physical fitness. However, they also noted that, because of inconsistent results among studies, there is currently insufficient evidence to assess the effectiveness of classroom-based health education focused on information provision, and health education classes focused on reducing TV viewing and video-game playing in increasing physical activity (Kahn et al., 2002). Furthermore, whilst school-based PE programmes appear to be successful in increasing activity during PE, there is limited evidence that they are effective in improving out-of-school physical activity levels.

Community-based interventions

Given that the majority of young people's physical activity occurs outside of school and that school-based programmes have had limited success in improving out-of-school activity, it would seem that programmes to complement school-based programmes are needed. As highlighted in Chapter 8, there is now increasing recognition of the importance of the involvement of the community at all levels if physical activity interventions are to be effective (Sallis, 1998). Despite this, reviews (e.g. Sallis et al., 1992; Sallis, 1998; Stone et al., 1998; Pate et al., 2000; Kahn et al., 2002) reveal relatively few community-based physical activity interventions with young people, and virtually all have been conducted in the US.

Reviews conducted by Sallis and colleagues (1992) and Sallis (1998) reported findings of a limited number of family-based intervention studies, but found no studies which had evaluated programmes in other community settings. The review conducted by Stone et al. (1998) considered both school- and community-based interventions which met specific inclusion criteria (see earlier), and identified only three completed community-based physical activity studies, and four which were in progress. Pate et al. (2000), meanwhile, reviewed just two studies. More recently, the systematic review of physical activity interventions conducted by Kahn et al. (2002) included 11 family-based intervention studies. These were broadly divided into those that were implemented as part of a school-based programme, such as CATCH and SPARK (highlighted earlier), and those that were implemented as independent studies in the community setting. Four independent studies were identified focusing on three interventions.

Intervention studies and findings

The Family Health Project (Nader et al., 1989) was an intensive nutrition and physical activity programme for families with preadolescents in San Diego. The intervention involved 206 families (including controls and intervention families), and targeted improvements in family support for healthful behaviours. The programme was found to be successful in increasing knowledge and changing dietary habits, but generally unsuccessful in increasing physical activity and fitness levels. The Center Based Program for Families (Baranowski et al., 1990) was a similar intensive programme with 94 African-American families, and involved education and fitness sessions based at a community centre. However, it was also found to be ineffective in increasing physical activity and fitness.

CATCH included a family component that consisted of take-home materials and Family Fun Night in-person sessions at the schools, designed to reinforce the school-based intervention. Nader et al. (1996) evaluated the family component and concluded that it resulted in improved knowledge and attitudinal effects, but did not influence behaviour change beyond that achieved through the school-based component.

In addition to programmes for healthy families, Sallis (1998) notes how several family-based programmes have been conducted with low-fit or obese children. For example, Taggart, Taggart & Siedentop (1986) conducted a 12-week programme with families of children with low fitness levels. Parents were taught to apply behaviour modification principles and to reward children's physical activity. All children increased both their activity and fitness levels, and some increased their activity levels over 100 per cent. Similarly, Epstein and colleagues have published the findings of a number of studies conducted with obese children. These were intensive clinical programmes undertaken by clinically obese children with at least one obese parent. Substantial and sustained reductions in percentage overweight were reported (Epstein et al., 1994).

Community-based interventions beyond the family level include the Minnesota Heart Health Program and the Class of 89 study (or Class of 89) (Kelder, Perry & Klepp, 1993) and Active Winners (Pate et al., 1997). The Class of 89 study involved over two thousand students and included both school and community intervention components. Physical activity was found to decline over time in both the intervention and control group, though the decline was smaller at all ages in the intervention group. Active Winners similarly encountered little success. The study was conducted with over two hundred primary- or elementary-aged youngsters who were predominantly rural African-American, and focused on increasing activity and fitness levels outside school. No significant changes in physical activity or physical fitness were found, though girls were reported to have significantly increased intentions to exercise.

Finally, one study, the initial evaluation of the Patient Centred Assessment and Counselling for Exercise plus Nutrition (PACE+) programme (Patrick et al., 2001), was found which had been conducted in the primary care setting. In PACE+, approximately a hundred and twenty adolescents completed a computerized assessment of their physical activity and nutrition behaviour and received counselling from their healthcare provider. They were then assigned to one of four types of intervention follow-up over a four-month period (no contact, frequent mail, infrequent mail and telephone, frequent mail and telephone). Results revealed that participants improved their moderate but not vigorous activity participation over time. No effect for follow-up condition was observed.

Thus, community-based physical activity intervention studies have produced equivocal results. Following their reviews, Sallis (1998) concluded that family-based programmes have been ineffective in increasing children's physical activity and cannot therefore be recommended for broad implementation, and Kahn et al. (2002) concluded that 'the available studies provide insufficient evidence to assess the effectiveness of family based social support interventions in increasing levels of physical activity or improving fitness, because of inconsistent results' (p. 84). Similarly, Stone et al. (1998) noted that the results provide limited positive findings. Despite this, Sallis (1998) summarized that there is strong potential for family-based interventions to be effective and Pate et al. (2000) concluded that there is some evidence for the feasibility of community approaches.

Trends, characteristics and issues in physical activity interventions

In analysing both the school- and community-based physical activity intervention studies, certain trends and characteristics are evident across both types of programmes. In addition, a number of issues come to light which should be of interest and relevance to PE teachers and health and other practitioners involved in planning, developing or implementing health-related or physical activity programmes with young people.

First, different types of school- and community-based programmes were evident. Broadly, the following types of school-based interventions were common:

1 Augmented PE programmes which involved lengthening the time of existing PE lessons or adding new or additional lessons.

2   Non-augmented or standard PE programmes which were incorporated into existing PE time. These involved increasing the amount of physical activity during lessons, for example, by changing the activities taught or modifying the rules of a game.
3   Classroom-based programmes which were based on theoretical instruction and the provision of information.

Most studies appeared to focus on augmented PE programmes which included the provision of additional PE time (Almond & Harris, 1998). However, given the pressures of curriculum time for PE, particularly in recent years (see Chapter 7), the feasibility and sustainability of such programmes for more widespread implementation is questionable.

With respect to the community interventions, the majority were at the family level (see Sallis, 1998; Kahn et al., 2002), though interventions had also been implemented in the wider community. Further, the target populations varied greatly. They included the low-fit or obese (e.g. Taggart, Taggart & Siedentop, 1986; Epstein et al., 1994), high-risk populations (e.g. Active Winners) and children from different ethnic groups (e.g. the Center Based Program for Families).

The collection of studies is largely from the US and limited to several age groups, with most of the studies having been conducted with upper-primary (elementary)-aged children (Stone et al., 1998). For example, the following school-based programmes (CATCH; Go for Health; the Nebraska School Study; the Southwest CV Curriculum Project; SPARK) and community-based programmes (Active Winners; the Center Based Program; the Family Health Project) were conducted with upper-primary-aged children. Just a minority of school-based studies (e.g. Slice of Life; the Stanford Adolescent Heart Health Program; Project Active Teens (Dale, Corbin & Cuddihy, 1988)) and community studies (e.g. Class of 89) have been conducted with older youth. Stone et al. (1998) suggest that the absence of preschool and early primary years in interventions is partially due to the difficulty in measuring physical activity as well as delivering interventions with these groups. Harris & Cale (1997), on the other hand, suggest that the predominance of primary school programmes may be due to the increased flexibility generally afforded by the primary curriculum and to their more holistic approach to health education. Also of interest is that far more school- than community-based intervention studies have been conducted. According to Sallis (1998), because community interventions can occur at different levels of influence, involve a wide range of individuals and organizations and use a variety of methods, they are difficult to plan, implement and evaluate. This may explain the relative dearth of community programmes.

Concerning the design and implementation of the interventions, the majority used random assignment experimental designs (e.g. CATCH; CHIC; the Center Based Program for Families; the Family Health Project; Slice of Life; the Southwest CV Curriculum Project), though some adopted quasi-experimental designs (non-randomized) (e.g. Active Winners; Class of 1989; Go for Health; SPARK; the Oslo Youth Study). CATCH is the first school-based, multicentre randomized trial ever conducted. Some researchers consider the use of random assignment and control groups a necessity in intervention research. Others, however, consider such experimental examinations an impossibility (Kemper, 1990). Tinning & Kirk (1991) highlight the limitations of adopting a scientifically-based, experimental approach within complex social settings such as schools (or communities). For example, they identified problems with the matching of control and experimental groups and with isolating the effects of programmes from control groups. Most studies, however, randomized or assigned schools, families or communities rather than individuals to intervention conditions. Given the complexities involved, though, in-depth, qualitative approaches to intervention research may have some merit.

For interventions to be critically evaluated, they require clearly defined and measurable goals that are based on the best available evidence defining valued outcomes. Physical activity interventions can influence physiological (physical fitness components such as aerobic capacity, muscular strength and endurance, flexibility), clinical (body composition, blood pressure, blood lipids), behavioural (physical activity and/or dietary behaviour), cognitive (knowledge and understanding about physical activity and/or exercise) and affective (attitudes) outcomes, and programme effectiveness can be gauged in terms of changes in any of these factors. The programmes reviewed here had varied aims and objectives and focused on a broad range of short-term outcomes. According to Stone et al. (1998), most school-based studies measured knowledge, attitudes and physical activity behaviour, most identified increasing levels of physical activity as a primary outcome, and a number also included fitness measures (e.g. CATCH; CHIC; the Nebraska School Study; the Oslo Youth Study; SPARK). Similarly, measures of physical activity and fitness were common in community-based studies (e.g. Active Winners; the Center Based Program for Families; the Family Health Project) and some also measured knowledge (e.g. the Family Health Project).

The emphasis by many studies on physiological outcomes such as the development of physical fitness is worthy of note. These typically involved the administration of fitness tests such as VO_2 max tests (e.g. CHIC; the Oslo Youth Study), a one mile run (the Nebraksa School Study), or a 9 minute run (CATCH). As the previous chapter revealed, there are a number of concerns and limitations concerning fitness tests with children, and the routine testing of children has been criticized on the grounds that it is 'archaic and inconsistent with our current understanding of the exercise-health connection' (Rowland, 1995, p. 125). For this and other reasons (see Chapter 9), it is argued that from a public health and physical activity promotion perspective, the goal should be to influence physical activity rather than fitness (Rowland, 1995; Pangrazi, 2000; Cale & Harris, 2002; Corbin, 2002), and that interventions should focus also on behavioural, cognitive and affective outcomes (Harris & Cale, 1997). Indeed, Shephard & Trudeau (2000) suggest that the ability of programmes to develop a habit of regular physical activity that persists throughout adult life seems more important than any short-term gains in fitness. Further, because the health benefits of physical activity in youth are transitory, it has been suggested that it is most important to establish patterns of regular participation in youth that can be carried into adulthood and to evaluate programme effectiveness on short- and long-term behavioural changes (Sallis et al., 1992; Pate et al., 2000; Richter et al., 2000). It would seem, though, that there needs to be consensus amongst researchers and practitioners alike concerning what health-related outcomes are valued most, and what physical activity interventions should be striving to achieve.

An encouraging theme in a number of the studies, and particularly within the school-based studies (e.g. CATCH; SPARK), was the use of multicomponent interventions versus a single-factor approach (Stone et al., 1998). Some of the components within the school-based programmes included intervening in the PE programme, the classroom curriculum, and with parents/families, as well as in out-of-school physical activity. It is logical to assume that interventions are likely to be most successful if they target the same behaviour across a number of levels. Most studies also addressed multiple behaviours, with diet being coupled most often with physical activity (Stone et al., 1998; Kahn et al., 2002). In addition, theoretical models were commonly used as a basis for the interventions, and a number of studies used a multiple theoretical approach (e.g. CATCH; Class of 89; the Oslo Youth Study; SPARK; the Southwest CV Curriculum Project). The most common theory was the Social

Cognitive Theory or Social Learning Theory, though others employed included Social Influences, Self-Monitoring, Cognitive Evaluation Theory (self-regulation) and Organizational Change Theory. See Chapter 6 for an overview of theoretical models of exercise motivation and behaviour change.

The interventions also varied greatly in size and duration. Ninety-six schools and 5106 students were involved in CATCH, whereas just one school and 270 students were involved in the Slice of Life Project. Almond & Harris (1998) identified a number of school-based studies with under a hundred students (e.g. MacConnie et al., 1982; Goldfine & Nahas, 1993; Ignico & Mahon, 1995). Sample sizes for community-based studies ranged from 200 youngsters (e.g. Active Winners) to over 2000 (e.g. Class of 89). In terms of the duration of the interventions, programmes ranged from just a few weeks or a term or two (e.g. 11 weeks for the Southwest CV Curriculum Project; 12 weeks for the Family Health Project; one semester for the Slice of Life Project; two semesters for Project Active Teens) to more than a year (e.g. 18 months for Active Winners; two years for the Nebraska School Study; the Oslo Youth Study; SPARK). Shephard & Trudeau (2000) note how the long-term effects of programmes have had little investigation. Follow-up has been carried out in only a minority of studies (Stone et al., 1998). Periods have included two months for the Stanford Adolescent Heart Project, one and a half years for SPARK, two years for the Family Health Project, three years for CATCH, seven years for Class of 89, 12 years for the Oslo Youth Study and 20+ years for the Trois Rivières study (Trudeau et al., 1998; 1999). Indeed, Shephard & Trudeau (2000) claim that the latter study represents the only experimental study examining the long-term impact of enhanced PE at the primary level. Given the short nature of many of the interventions and the lack of longitudinal designs, it is perhaps not surprising that equivocal findings or no significant changes have been reported in some instances. Further, the available evidence from long-term evaluations suggests that the long-term effects of programmes remain rather weak (Shephard & Trudeau, 2000). Additional longitudinal studies are clearly required.

With the community-based studies, further reasons have also been proposed to account for the equivocal findings. For example, some studies encountered problems with attrition and obtaining family participation in the interventions (Sallis, 1998). In the Center Based Program for Families, participation rates were only 20 per cent and during the maintenance phase of the Family Health Project, attendance was approximately 40 per cent. Thus, increasing participation rates in family programmes would seem to be a critical challenge (Sallis, 1998). On this issue, Stone et al. (1998) suggest that a reduction of barriers in high-risk groups in particular needs careful planning to optimize recruitment and participation. In the CATCH programme, meanwhile, the authors suggested that the lack of specific behaviour change may have been the result of the low intensity of the home-based intervention (Nader et al., 1996). An interesting finding with the family programmes, however, is that, despite their ineffectiveness for healthy populations, they appear to be effective among low-fit or obese populations. Overall, it would seem that greater understanding is needed about the family as a unit for intervention.

On the whole, the studies provided limited detail regarding the specific intervention protocols employed. This makes the replication of studies difficult and provides little direction or guidance for the future development of studies, interventions and practice. Furthermore, and in the case of the school-based programmes, it has been suggested that where the content was outlined it did not appear to be especially innovative or to include the type of physical activity which would appeal to many young people (Cale & Harris, 1998). For example, programmes included aerobic conditioning techniques or timed runs, and many others were based on theoretical classroom instruction (Cale & Harris, 1998). Although the former activities may positively influence short-term fitness gains, they may not be so successful in promoting lifetime physical activity (Harris & Cale, 1997). Similarly, Harris & Elbourn (1992) argue that sedentary classroom-based delivery of health-related concepts is limited in that it tends to focus on information transmission rather than the essential combination of understanding, experiencing, decision-making and evaluating. This could in part explain why such programmes have been found to be relatively ineffective.

Of course, programme content must also be considered in the light of the desired outcomes. Thus, if the desired outcome is 'lifelong physical activity', then the content must reflect this goal and should focus on the development of activities and skills 'that promote generalization and maintenance of physical activity during youth and adolescence and enhance the probability of carryover to adulthood' (Sallis et al., 1992, p. S255). This may require a focus on more individually oriented and unstructured activity which is more characteristic of adult physical activity. Given the strong emphasis of schools' PE curricula on competitive sports and team games, however (Penney & Evans, 1999; Fairclough, Stratton & Baldwin, 2002) (see Chapter 7), this is likely to present a particular challenge for school-based programmes.

Also evident from the reviews and the studies is that, generally, a limited range of physical activity interventions have been applied to young people. Most studies addressed more than one component but the majority targeted the individual and ignored potentially important environmental factors. This issue is also raised in Chapters 4 and 8. To date, little research has examined these effects on youth (Richter et al., 2000; Wechsler et al., 2000). Resnicow, Robinson & Frank (1996), however, highlight the need to examine how the individual and the environment interact to influence behaviour. The importance of the whole-school environment in influencing young people's physical activity was highlighted in Chapters 4 and 7. Yet, and as acknowledged in these earlier chapters, school-based studies have primarily been limited to changes in the curriculum as opposed to whole-school policies or to the environment (Wechsler et al., 2000; Fox & Harris, 2003). Limited data on the contribution of school environmental factors to the physical activity levels of young people has been found (Wechsler et al., 2000). Currently, the Middle School Physical Activity and Nutrition (M-Span) project (McKenzie, 2001) is investigating whether school environmental changes can lead to improved physical activity and dietary habits in children and may provide some insight into this issue.

Similarly, in terms of developing community interventions, Sallis (1998) suggests that it is useful to apply ecological models of health behaviour which recognize the multiple influences on health-related physical activity. In addition, other community settings and approaches may have potential with young people. The review by Kahn et al. (2002), for example, revealed a range of interventions which have been found to be effective in increasing levels of physical activity in adults (e.g. point-of-decision prompts, social support interventions in community settings, individually adapted health behaviour change programmes, the creation of or enhanced access to places for physical activity), yet which have largely been unexplored with young people. Likewise, the initial positive findings from PACE+ (Patrick et al., 2001), coupled with examples of effective physical activity interventions with adults (Sallis et al., 2000), suggest that the primary care setting provides scope for promoting physical activity with young people. A recent review of physical activity (and nutrition) interventions for youth in primary care (Sallis et al., 2000) revealed no published studies of such interventions for young people.

Kahn et al. (2002) highlight the role of multisite, multicomponent interventions in successfully increasing physical activity behaviours, and it is encouraging to see that the designs and strategies used in the more recent intervention studies include more randomized trials, involve multicomponent interventions and often address measurement of multiple behaviours and environmental behaviours (Stone et al., 1998). However, although these approaches are favoured in that they are more likely to capture the range of influences on young people's physical activity, there are difficulties in evaluation in teasing out the specific effects on physical activity, and deciding which strategies are most effective, and which factors or aspects of an intervention determine success (Fox & Harris, 2003).

Summary of physical activity interventions

In summary, it would seem that school-based PE programmes can provide encouraging results and be effective in increasing young people's physical activity and fitness. Community-based programmes have had limited success, however, and the findings from studies are equivocal. The research base for physical activity intervention studies is still relatively sparse and is limited for community-based studies in particular. Few studies have been conducted outside the US and, owing to a lack of longitudinal research, the long-term effects of programmes remain unknown. Furthermore, studies have primarily targeted the individual rather than the environment and there would appear to be ample scope for developing a broader range of approaches and multilevel interventions with young people. On the basis of the evidence from school-based intervention studies, Fox & Harris (2003) concluded that the existing literature is not sufficiently extensive to provide definitive guidelines for schools about which types or aspects of programmes are most effective in promoting activity. The same can certainly also be concluded for community-based studies and guidance for health and other professionals working in community settings.

Discussion point   Taking into account what you have read within this and earlier chapters (see Chapters 7 and 8 in particular), what recommendations do you feel could be made to physical educators and health professionals for future school- and/or community-based physical activity intervention practice?

Physical activity promotion initiatives

Increasingly, government, commercial organizations and charitable trusts are supporting the promotion and development of sports and physical activity opportunities for young people. Outlined here are a number of government and non-government national UK school- and community-based physical activity initiatives which are relevant to young people. The list is far from exhaustive but aims to cover some of the key initiatives, as well as reflect the range of initiatives available. Other community-based initiatives which have been employed with or are relevant to young people are highlighted in Chapter 8. Unless otherwise stated, the information presented has been accessed from the relevant organizations' web sites (see Table 10.4 for details).

Government strategies and associated initiatives

The Sports Strategy

The Government's most recent sports strategy, *A Sporting Future for All* (DCMS, 2001), proposed a five-part plan to increase participation in sport by young people through improving the quantity and quality of PE and sport provision in schools. The plan proposed to allocate 20 per cent of lottery funds to youth sport, the bulk of which would be spent in schools, and to commit funding to improve sport facilities in primary schools, extend the Specialist Sports Colleges and School Sport Co-ordinators programmes, support schools to provide out-of-school-hours learning opportunities including PE and sport, and to improve provision for talented youngsters.

The PE, School Sport and Club Links Strategy

More recently still, the government has shown an even greater commitment to PE and sport in schools with the launch of the PE, School Sport and Club Links Strategy. As acknowledged in Chapter 7, the strategy was launched in October 2002 and is being supported by a government investment of £459 million over three years. The aim is to increase the percentage of schoolchildren in England who spend a minimum of two hours each week in high-quality PE and school sport within and beyond the curriculum from 25 per cent in 2002, to 75 per cent by 2006 (DfES, 2003). The strategy is being delivered by the DfES and DCMS through eight programmes (a description of four of such programmes follows): Specialist Sports Colleges; School Sport Co-ordinators (SSCos); Gifted and Talented; QCA PE and School Sport Investigation; Step into Sport; Professional Development; School/Club Links; and Swimming.

Specialist Sports Colleges   Specialist Sports Colleges were introduced in 1997 as part of the Specialist Schools Programme run by the

Department for Education and Skills (DfES). Any maintained secondary school in England may apply to become a Specialist School but to be designated must meet certain conditions. In return, they receive additional capital and funding (DfES, 2002). As of March 2002, there were 141 designated Sports Colleges, with a latest government target of 400 by September 2005 (DfES, 2003). The specific aims of Sports Colleges are:

- To raise standards of achievement in PE and sport through the increased quality of teaching and learning.
- To extend and enrich curriculum and out-of-hours learning opportunities in PE and sport.
- To increase take-up and interest in PE and other sporting or physical activity related courses, particularly post-16.
- To raise standards by developing good practice and disseminating and sharing with other schools and groups, including non-specialist secondary schools.
- To work with appropriate local partners, including business and community groups, clubs, governing bodies and sports development units, to develop sustainable sporting opportunities which promote both participation and achievement in PE and community sport. (DfES, 2001)

The School Sport Co-ordinator (SSCo) Programme The School Sport Co-ordinator Programme was introduced in September 2000 and is a multi-agency initiative involving the DfES, DCMS, Sport England, the NOF (New Opportunities Fund) and the YST (Youth Sport Trust). The programme focuses on communities of greatest need and involves families of schools working together to enhance sports opportunities for all. Partnerships are usually made up of a Specialist Sports College, eight secondary schools and around forty-five primary schools, with each partnership receiving up to £270,000 per year (DfES, 2003). The funding supports a professional development manager for each partnership, SSCos (school sport co-ordinators), usually experienced teachers who are released from the timetable two days a week to co-ordinate and drive development in each family of schools, plus PLTs (primary link teachers). Six strategic objectives have been set for SSCo partnerships:

- Strategic planning – develop and implement a PE/sport strategy
- Primary liaison – develop links
- Out-of-school hours – provide enhanced opportunities for all pupils

- School to community – increase participation in community sport
- Coaching and leadership – provide opportunities for senior pupils, teachers and other adults
- Raising standards – of pupils' achievement (DfES, 2003)

As of September 2002, there were 146 partnerships, with 750 SSCos, with an ultimate government target of 400 partnerships, 3200 SSCos and 18,000 PLTs by September 2006 (DfES, 2003; YST, 2002).

Step into Sport   Step into Sport is a programme which encourages children, young people and adults to begin and continue an involvement in sports leadership and volunteering. In addition, it encourages governing bodies, county sports partnerships and clubs to develop and implement volunteering strategies. In this way, it aims to ensure that local clubs are prepared to receive, develop and deploy a steady supply of new volunteers. From 2002–04 the programme is being delivered in up to two hundred SSCo partnerships by a consortium of the YST, the British Sports Trust and Sport England.

School/Club Links   The School/Club Links programme aims to build on and enhance the existing PE and sport opportunities available to young people in schools and thereby increase the proportion of children guided into clubs from SSCo partnerships by guiding them from schools to National Governing Body (NGB) affiliated or otherwise accredited clubs linked to those partnerships. The project focuses on seven major sports (tennis, cricket, rugby union, football, athletics, gymnastics and swimming), though links to a broader range of sports and physical activity are also encouraged. The key partners at national level are the DCMS, Sport England, the YST and the NGBs of the seven sports.

Sport England and associated initiatives

Sport England has been, and continues to be, instrumental in supporting the development of sport and physical activity opportunities for young people. For example, Sport England's former Active programmes – Active Schools, Active Communities and Active Sports – each comprised initiatives that were relevant to young people. A selection of Active Schools and Active Communities initiatives is presented in Tables 10.1 and 10.2.

Active England   More recently, Sport England is striving 'to get 70 per cent of the population doing 30 minutes of activity a day by

Table 10.1 Example Active Schools initiatives

Product/Service	Aims	Features
Activemark/Activemark Gold	To recognize and reward a school for its commitment to providing quality physical activity provision.	A recognition and reward scheme for outstanding physical activity programmes. An auditing and development tool.
Sportsmark/Sportsmark Gold	To recognize and reward a school for its commitment to providing quality PE and school sport provision.	A recognition and reward scheme for outstanding PE and school sport programmes. An auditing and development tool.
Coaching for Teachers	To enable teachers to provide a wider range of out-of-school-hours activities.	A joint Sport England and Sports Coach UK initiative. Low-cost access to coaching courses in a wide range of activities to update and develop coaching skills.
Awards for All	To develop school/club links and out-of-hours learning opportunities.	One-off grants from £500 to £5000 to develop links with local sports clubs and enhance out-of-hours provision.

Sporting Champions	To inspire and motivate young people to participate in sport.	Sporting heroes/heroines visit schools, youth and sports clubs to encourage young people to take part.
Sportsearch	To help young people to identify and fulfil their sporting potential.	An internet CD-ROM system to help young people make informed choices about sport. Signposts suitable sports/places to take part locally.
Primary Sports Day Toolkit	To enable primary school teachers to co-ordinate and deliver inclusive and active sports days.	A pack full of practical ideas to help run an active, inclusive and fun sports day. A focus on generic skill development.
Active Kids' Clubs	To help Kids' Clubs develop physical activity and sport.	A joint initiative between Sport England and KCN (Kids' Clubs Network), the national childcare charity. A funded post to develop physical activity programmes for Kids' Clubs. Training, activity programmes and resources to support child care workers.

Table 10.2   Example Active Communities initiatives

Service/Product/ Funding	Aims	Features
Positive Futures	To use sport to reduce antisocial behaviour, crime and drug misuse among 10–16 year olds within local neighbourhoods.	A partnership between Sports England, the UK Anti Drugs Coordination Unit and the Youth Justice Board. Projects involved a sporting activity programme, an inclusion programme, self-awareness and drug prevention, and an education and training programme.
Community Small Projects: Awards for All	To develop sports or activity opportunities in the community in order to extend access and participation, increase skills and creativity, and improve quality of life.	Grants from £500 to £5000 for local groups, schools, health bodies to develop new or existing sports or activity opportunities in the community.
GirlSport	To enhance communication and understanding of the issues that affect teenage girls' enjoyment, involvement and progress in sport and physical activity.	Encouraged teenagers and adults to share ideas and problems, and generate solutions to the challenges girls face in participation. An interactive workshop and a *GirlSport* magazine.

2020' (www.sportemgland.org/active/ae). Active England is a joint £108.5 million community sport investment programme from the Sport England and the New Opportunities Fund that supports a number of innovative projects that demonstrate the ability to work towards this target. The Active England fund seeks to create and support sustainable innovative multi-activity environments in areas of social, sport and health deprivation, and to increase participation among all sections of society.

Sportsmatch Sportsmatch is funded by the DCMS through grant aid from Sport England and administered by the Institute of Sports Sponsorship. It is a grass-roots sports sponsorship incentive scheme open to any non-profit-making group such as a school, college, sports club, governing body or local authority. Pound for pound, it can match commercial business sponsorship for a grass-roots sporting event or activity and acts as an incentive by offering to double the pot of money available from a sponsor. Girls, schools and youth are amongst the priority groups for this award.

The Healthy Schools Programme
The Healthy Schools Programme is jointly run by the DoH and the DfES. As highlighted in Chapter 7, the programme was launched in 1998 and aims to raise awareness of the opportunities in schools for improving health, both physical and mental, of children and teachers, as well as of families and the local community. It encourages schools to develop a 'healthy school' ethos and to develop and improve school and community links. The programme has a national network – the Wired for Health website (www.wiredforhealth.gov.uk). Every local education authority in England is working in partnership with primary care trusts to manage a local Healthy Schools Programme. The local programmes provide support to schools to help them become healthy and effective, and each has a local co-ordinator and a team from education and health supporting its management and delivery. Other components of the Healthy Schools Programme include the NHSS (National Healthy School Standard), which provides national quality standards for local Healthy Schools Programmes, and a National Healthy Schools Newsletter, which provides information on the NHSS, and updates on the Healthy Schools Programme and related activities/initiatives. Physical activity is a specific theme within the NHSS.

STAG (the School Travel Advisory Group)
Developed in conjunction with the DTLR (Department for Transport, Local Government and the Regions), STAG aims to raise the profile of school travel issues and reduce car journeys to school where safer, healthy alternatives exist. It identifies practical ways of reducing car use and

ensures that policy and initiatives affecting school travel are integrated across transport, health and education.

Non-government initiatives

Safe Routes to School

Safe Routes to School is an initiative developed by Sustrans, the sustainable transport charity (see Chapter 8). It is a community approach to encouraging and enabling more people to walk or cycle to school through a combined package of practical and educational measures. The initiative also strives to improve road safety and reduce child casualties, improve children's health and development, and reduce traffic congestion and pollution. Example projects include introducing school safety zones with 20 mph speed limits, walking buses, safe cycle storage or lockers for cyclists/pedestrians, cycle or pedestrian training, and 'walk to school' or 'road safety' weeks.

Home Zones

Home Zones is a Children's Play Council initiative. Home Zones are streets designed primarily to meet the interests of, and be more attractive to pedestrians and cyclists rather than motorists by, for example, introducing traffic calming, parking areas, trees and bushes, benches or play areas to slow traffic down. Pilot Home Zone projects supported by the DTLR are currently under way.

The Neighbourhood Play Toolkit

Another initiative developed by the Children's Play Council is the Neighbourhood Play Toolkit. This is a three-year project which aims to develop a comprehensive pack for supporting the strategic development of play space. Resources will be published as a comprehensive 'neighbourhood play toolkit', which will lead stakeholders through a community-based participative process for identifying and implementing change and improvement to play spaces.

TOP Programmes

The TOP Programmes have been developed by the YST and are a series of linked and progressive schemes for all young people aged 18 months to 18 years. The programmes form a sporting pathway along which young people can progress according to their age and development. Resource cards, child-friendly equipment and quality training and support for teachers and deliverers are key features of the TOP programmes. Programmes include TOP Tots, TOP Start, TOP Play, TOP Sport, TOP Skill, TOP Link and TOP Sportsability.

Zoneparc

This is a playground improvement project also developed by the YST and supported by the DfES and Nike. The initiative involves introducing innovative break-time activities in an attempt to tackle social exclusion and increase primary children's physical activity levels. Play equipment and resources, plus training for break-time supervisors and support staff are provided and a number of pupils are appointed as Zoneparc players to help organize activities in the playground.

Jump Rope for Heart

Jump Rope for Heart is a BHF (British Heart Foundation)-sponsored skipping challenge. It aims to promote healthy exercise among young people, raise funds for the BHF and the schools or groups taking part, and encourage teachers to develop physical activity opportunities. Schools or groups who register for the initiative receive an organizer's kit, comprising skipping ropes and other materials, as well as a teachers' pack that provides activity ideas. An optional workshop is also offered to teachers/leaders.

Midnight Basketball

Midnight Basketball is managed and organized by the NPFA (National Playing Fields Association) and delivered locally through a network of partnerships with targeted agencies such as the youth and community services, sports development departments, the police, probation service, social services and youth offending teams. It aims to support the learning needs of young people and encourage them to participate in mainstream society, provide a safe and positive environment, and divert young people from crime, antisocial behaviour and drug, alcohol and other physical abuse. The programme consists of 12 sessions which comprise an educational workshop covering topics such as citizenship, drugs awareness and sexual health, plus basketball activities.

Youth Moves

Youth Moves is a KFA (Keep Fit Association) initiative for 4–16-year-olds which aims to stimulate creativity and fitness through fun, safe, friendly and non-competitive movement, exercise and dance classes.

Sessions are taken by qualified KFA teachers who have been trained to work with young people.

Nike GIS (Girls in Sport) Project

The GIS project is a partnership between Nike, the YST and teachers, and was established in 1999 with the aim of encouraging more 11–14-year-olds girls to take part enthusiastically in PE and sport (Kirk et al., 2000; O'Donovan, 2002). It comprises a training course for PE staff and pupils, a manual for each school, and assistance in developing an action plan focusing on changing aspects of PE and sport policy, delivery and provision.

Discussion point　　Organizations and initiatives at regional and local level can also support the promotion of physical activity.

Which local organizations or partners could support the promotion of physical activity among young people in your area?

Are you aware of any local programmes and initiatives that support the promotion of physical activity in young people? If so, which?

Resources and contacts

Summarized in Tables 10.3 and 10.4 are a list of resources and contacts which may further assist in the promotion of physical activity in young people. The lists are by no means exhaustive. The selection of resources has been made based on their relevance either to the National Curriculum or to physical activity promotion practice, and in terms of their consistency with the key messages and philosophy advocated throughout this text.

Discussion of initiatives, resources and contacts

As can be seen, there has been a great deal of activity by government departments and other organizations in terms of developing policy, initiatives and resources to promote and develop sports and physical activity opportunities for young people. The PE, School Sport and Club Links Strategy is the first national strategy of its kind and represents the largest financial investment in PE and school sport ever made by government. In addition, the number and range of other initiatives and organizations involved is impressive and suggests a serious and widespread commitment and interest in young people's physical activity participation. However, a few points concerning such activity are worthy of note.

Table 10.3 Physical activity promotion resources

Resource	Key Stage (KS) (where applicable)	Description	Available from:
Health-Related Exercise in the National Curriculum (Harris (2000))	1–4	Teacher Training Agency kitemarked guidance material for HRE covering terminology, rationale, recommendations, delivery, assessment, National Curriculum requirements, and approaches. It also contains a scheme and units of work, resources and contacts.	Human Kinetics, Leeds; 0113 278 1708; hk@hkeurope.com
Health-Related Exercise Posters (ACCAC/FBA & Harris (1996))	1–4	A set of 4 laminated colour posters (A1 size) for KS1 & 2 and 7 laminated colour posters (A1 size) for KS3 & 4 containing key health and fitness messages and information.	FBA, 4 The Science Park, Aberystwyth, Ceredigion, SY23 3AH; 01970 611996
Warming Up and Cooling Down (Harris & Elbourn (2002))	1–4	A text which addresses the knowledge base/theory of warming up and cooling down and provides practical ideas and examples in a range of National Curriculum activities.	Human Kinetics, Leeds; 0113 278 1708; hk@hkeurope.com

Table 10.3 (Continued)

Resource	Key Stage (KS) (where applicable)	Description	Available from:
The Active School Resource Packs for Primary or Secondary Schools (British Heart Foundation (2000))	1–4	Packs aimed at primary or secondary teachers which contain information on the aims and philosophy of an Active School, developing a physical activity policy and development plan, plus practical ideas and activity cards, resources and contacts.	British Heart Foundation, c/o Peterhurst Ltd, 262 Water Road, Wembley, Middlesex, HA0 IWB (order form can be downloaded from http://www.bhf.org.uk/youngpeople)
Getting it Right. The Y's Guide to Safe and Effective Exercise (London Central YMCA (1994))	1–4	A 40-minute video (+booklet) which covers warming up and cooling down, stamina, strength and suppleness training, exercise appraisal, and includes PE, sport and exercise examples.	YMCA Fitness Industry Training, 111 Great Russell Street, London, WC1B 3NP; 020 7343 1850
Teaching Health-Related Exercise at Key Stages 1 and 2 (Harris & Elbourn (1997))	1–2	A text which covers children and exercise, safe exercise, National Curriculum requirements, and whole-school approaches to physical activity promotion. It also provides example lessons and practical activities.	Human Kinetics, Leeds; 0113 278 1708; hk@hkeurope.com

Resource		Description	Contact
Health-Related Exercise at Key Stage 3. Resource Pack for Pupils and Teachers (ACCAC/FBA & Harris (2000))	3	An A4 ring binder resource comprising 10 laminated pupil task cards and a teacher's handbook addressing the HRE requirements of the KS3 National Curriculum.	FBA, 4 The Science Park, Aberystwyth, Ceredigion, SY23 3AH; 01970 636400
'Fit for Life' Health-Related Exercise at Key Stage 4 (Harris & Cale (2001)) Loughborough University and the Youth Sport Trust	4	A file comprising 21 pupil task cards and a teachers' handbook addressing the HRE requirements of the KS4 National Curriculum.	The Youth Sport Trust, Sir John Beckwith Centre for Sport, Loughborough University, Loughborough, LE11 3TU; 01509 226600; ystinfo@lboro.ac.uk
Planning a Personal Exercise Programme (Elbourn & YMCA Fitness Industry Training (1998))	4	A manual comprising 12 practical session plans which help young people to build the skills, knowledge and understanding associated with planning, monitoring and evaluating a personal exercise programme.	CYMCA Qualifications, 111 Great Russell Street, London, WC1B 3NP; 0171 343 1800
Assisting a Circuit Training Instructor (Elbourn, Brennan & YMCA Fitness Industry Training (1998))	4	A manual comprising 10 practical session plans which build the skills, knowledge and understanding necessary to assist a qualified fitness instructor in planning, delivering and evaluating circuit classes.	CYMCA Qualifications, 111 Great Russell Street, London, WC1B 3NP; 0171 343 1800

Table 10.3 (Continued)

Resource	Key Stage (KS) (where applicable)	Description	Available from:
Assisting an Exercise to Music Instructor (Elbourn, Brennan & YMCA Fitness Industry Training (1998))	4	A manual comprising 10 practical session plans which build the skills, knowledge and understanding necessary to assist a qualified fitness instructor in planning, delivering and evaluating exercise to music classes.	CYMCA Qualifications, 111 Great Russell Street, London, WC1B 3NP; 0171 343 1800
Aerobics and Circuits at Key Stage 4 (Elbourn (2002))	4	This manual comprises 26 progressive learning activities and a free CD containing over 100 printable circuit cards.	Coachwise Limited; 0113 201 5555; www.1st4sport.com
Aerobics and Circuits at Key Stage 4 Videos (2002)	4	These 45-minute videos demonstrate a range of practical ideas for using aerobics and circuits as contexts for learning. The videos also include useful clips of correct technique for a range of exercises.	Coachwise Limited; 0113 201 5555; www.1st4sport.com
Fitness Room Activities in Secondary Schools (Elbourn (2004))	4	This manual comprises 30 progressive learning activities and a free CD containing over 140 printable circuit cards.	CYMCA Qualifications, 111 Great Russell Street, London, WC1B 3NP; 0171 343 1800

Title		Description	Source
Young People and Physical Activity: A Guide to Resources (HDA (1999))		A guide which provides an overview of the national resources and programmes available to help professionals promote physical activity to young people.	Health Development Agency, PO Box 90, Wetherby, Yorkshire, LS23 7EX; 0870 121 4194
National Healthy School Standard (NHSS): Physical Activity (DoH & DfEE (2000))		This is support material which illustrates how local programme co-ordinators might address the physical activity components of the NHSS.	Health Development Agency, PO Box90, Wetherby, Yorkshire, LS23 7EX; 0870 121 4194. Can also be downloaded from www.wiredforhealth.gov.uk/healthy/ physical_activity_report_v.pdf
Young and Active? Young People and Health-Enhancing Physical Activity—Evidence and Implications (Biddle, Sallis & Cavill (eds) (1998))		A text which presents a policy framework for young people and physical activity, plus scientific review papers, recommendations for key agencies, and physical activity guidelines for young people.	Health Development Agency, PO Box 90, Wetherby, Yorkshire, LS23 7EX; 0870 121 4194
Guidance on Safe Active Travel to School in Primary Teacher Training (HDA (2000))	1–2	This resource provides guidance on issues relating to safe active travel to school including health-enhancing physical activity, direct health impacts of road transport, transport issues, and school-related issues.	Health Development Agency, PO Box 90, Wetherby, Yorkshire, LS23 7EX; 0870 121 4194. Also available from www.wiredforhealth.gov.uk/ new/safetrav.pdf

Table 10.3 (Continued)

Resource	Key Stage (KS) (where applicable)	Description	Available from:
Healthy Active Travel	1–4	This is a database of classroom materials relating to healthy, active travel. It provides a catalogue of information and resources relating to encouraging greater use of walking, cycling, public transport and car sharing for school journeys.	The database is available at www.databases.detr.gov.uk/schools/
School Travel Resource Pack	1–4	This pack contains photocopiable material for anyone involved in developing school strategies and plans. It provides information on the benefits of a school travel plan, the school journey, traffic congestion and pollution, health and fitness, etc.	Available at www.local-transport.detr.gov.uk/schooltravel/respack/index.htm
Home Zones: A Planning and Design Handbook (Children's Play Council (2001))		A handbook reviewing the evolution of Home Zones and the practical lessons emerging from the pilot schemes. Relevant for anyone interested in planning and designing a Home Zone.	Can be ordered from homezones@ncb.org.uk

First, the majority of initiatives, and particularly those emanating from government policy (e.g. the Sports Strategy; the PE, School Sport and Club Links Strategy; Sport England's programmes), focus on the promotion and development of 'sport' and 'sporting opportunities' for young people. By contrast, only a minority appear to promote lifetime physical activity and focus on lifestyle and unstructured or recreational activities (e.g. Safe Routes to School; Home Zones; the Neighbourhood Play Toolkit; Zoneparc). Indeed, Green (2002) and Penney & Evans (1999) have commented on how government appears to view sport, and particularly team games, as the primary vehicle for the promotion of ongoing involvement in health-promoting, active lifestyles. It could be argued that these initiatives are unlikely to be attractive to, and therefore benefit and meet the needs of, all young people. This argument was also levelled at the PE curriculum in Chapter 7. Clearly, the Professional Development programme within the PE, School Sport and Club Links Strategy (DfES, 2003) has the potential to address this issue and it is hoped that it will be instrumental in influencing developments in this respect.

Also, whilst the amount of activity should be applauded, to date much of it has appeared rather fragmented. It seems that teachers, health and other professionals have been bombarded with initiatives and resources, with little guidance on how to select, manage, co-ordinate and evaluate them to meet specific objectives and needs, or to translate them into meaningful, relevant and educational physical activity experiences and provision for young people. Indeed, in an article focusing on the work of Sport England and their former Active Schools programmes, Hendley (2003) asked whether such programmes represented 'high impact' or 'initiative overload?' Thus it would seem that there is a need for greater co-ordination of effort across a range of partners. Indeed, working in partnership is a recurring theme within the recommendations developed by the HEA (1998) for agencies and organizations with a role to play in promoting physical activity for young people. There are some good examples of collaboration and co-ordination of initiatives (e.g. the Healthy Schools Programme), but in many instances it seems that partnership opportunities have not been capitalized on. Significant progress in this area should, however, soon be seen with the implementation of the PE, School Sport and Club Links Strategy which is based on a strategic and co-ordinated approach. Its delivery is being overseen by a project board comprising representatives from various organizations (e.g. schools, the PE associations, YST, Sport England, government departments, NGBs), and one of the key targets is to establish a national infrastructure for PE and school sport (DfES, 2003).

Also on a positive note, the HEA (1998) recommends that programmes should be designed to meet the specific needs of young people and differentiated on the grounds of gender, age/life-stage and socio-economic status. It is therefore encouraging to see that some initiatives are differentiated and have been designed to meet the needs of specific groups. Examples include those targeted at girls (e.g. the Nike GIS Project), youngsters at risk (e.g. Midnight Basketball) and communities of greatest need (e.g. the SSCo programme).

Finally, unlike the formally evaluated school- and community-based interventions which were highlighted earlier, only a minority of these initiatives have or will be subjected to rigorous evaluation. Notable exceptions include the programmes that form part of the PE, School Sport and Clubs Links Strategy (e.g. the Specialist Sports Colleges initiative (Penney, Houlihan & Eley, 2002)) and the Nike GIS project (O'Donovan, 2002). However, owing to a lack of or limited evaluation, little is known about the effectiveness of many potentially valuable initiatives such as Home Zones, Safe Routes to School, or their respective elements such as 'walking buses', new cycle routes, traffic reduction/calming schemes, or the ways in which each of these influence the lifestyles of children (Fox & Harris, 2003). Fox & Harris (2003) suggest that until such an evidence base is constructed, the design and delivery of effective activity promotion initiatives will remain uninformed, undirected and sporadic. Likewise, the impact or likely impact of the resources available is largely unknown. The limitations of curriculum resources generally in initiating 'real' change have been acknowledged (Darling-Hammond, 1990; Sparkes, 1991; Capel, 2000). Cale, Harris & Leggett (2002) evaluated the impact of one health-related exercise resource (Harris, 2000) on secondary school PE teachers and found it to have a positive impact on aspects of policy and practice in a significant number of schools, but to be less successful in influencing deeper-level changes (e.g. in teaching philosophy and teaching styles). Studies of this nature, however, are rare.

Activity

Access a selection of the web sites for the organizations listed in Table 10.4. From the information provided, consider how each organization may be able to support physical educators, health professionals or other practitioners in the promotion of physical activity in young people? What service(s) does the organization provide and how might these make a difference?

Table 10.4 Useful contacts

Organization	Address	Tel nos/e-mail	Web site
British Heart Foundation (BHF)	Education Department, 14 Fitzhardinge Street, London W1H 6DH	020 7935 0185 Jump Rope for Heart – 020 7487 7149	www.bhf.org.uk
BHF National Centre for Physical Activity and Health	School of Sport and Exercise Sciences, Loughborough University, Loughborough LE11 3TU	01509 223259 bhfactive@lists. lboro.ac.uk	www.bhfactive.org.uk/index.htm
British Sports Trust	Clyde House, 10 Milburn Avenue, Oldbrook, Milton Keynes MK6 2WA	01908 689180 info@bst.org.uk	www.bst.org.uk
Children's Play Council	National Children's Bureau, 8 Wakley Street, London EC1V 7QE	020 7843 6016 cpc@ncb.org.uk	www.ncb.org.uk/cpc/
English Federation of Disability Sport	Manchester Metropolitan University, Hassall Road, Alsager, Stoke on Trent ST7 2HL	0161 247 5294 federation@efds.co.uk	www.efds.net
Health Development Agency	Holborn Gate, 330 High Holborn, London WC1V 7BA	020 7430 0850 communications@ hda-online.org.uk	www.hda-online.org.uk
Institute of Youth Sport	Sir John Beckwith Centre for Sport, Loughborough University, Loughborough LE11 3TU	01509 228410	www.lboro.ac.uk/departments/sses/institutes/iys
Keep Fit Association	Astra House, Suite 1.05, Arklow Road, London SE14 6EB	020 8692 9566 kfa@keepfit.org.uk	www.keepfit.org.uk
National Playing Fields Association	Head Office, Stanley House, St Chad's Place, London WC1X 9HH	020 7833 5360 npfa@npfa.co.uk	www.npfa.co.uk

Table 10.4   (Continued)

Organization	Address	Tel nos/e-mail	Web site
Physical Education Association of the United Kingdom	Ling House, Building 25, London Road, Reading RG1 5AQ	0118 931 6240 enquiries@pea.uk.com	www.pea.uk.com
Sports Coach UK	114 Cardigan Road, Headingley, Leeds LS6 3BJ	0113 274 4802 coaching@ sportscoachuk.org	www.sportscoachuk. org
Sport England	3rd Floor, Victoria House, Bloomsbury Square, London WC1B 4SE	08458 508508 info@sportengland.org	www.sportengland.org
Sustrans	Head Office, 35 King Street, Bristol BS1 4DZ	0117 926 8893 Project info – 0117 929 0888 Safe Routes to Schools – 0117 915 0100 info@sustrans.org.uk	www.sustrans.org.uk
Women's Sports Foundation	3rd Floor, Victoria House, Bloomsbury Square, London WC1B 4SE	020 7273 1740 info@wsf.org.uk	www.wsf.org.uk
Youth Sport Trust	Sir John Beckwith Centre for Sport, Loughborough University, Loughborough LE11 3TU	01509 226600 ystinfo@lboro.ac.uk	www.youthsporttrust.org
YMCA Fitness Industry Training	111 Great Russell Street, London WC1B 3NP	020 7343 1850 info@ymcafit.org.uk	www.ymcafit.org.uk
CYMCA Qualifications	As above	020 7343 1800	

References

Almond, L. & Harris, J. (1998) Interventions to promote health-related physical education. In Biddle, S., Sallis, J. & Cavill, N. (eds), *Young and Active? Young People and Health-Enhancing Physical Activity – Evidence and Implications*. London: HEA, 133–49.

Baranowski, T., Simons-Morton, B., Hooks, P., Henske, J., Tiernan, K. et al. (1990) A center-based program for exercise change among black-American families, *Health Education Quarterly*, **17**, 179–96.

Cale, L. & Harris, J. (1998) The benefits of health-related physical education and recommendations for implementation, *The Bulletin of Physical Education*, **34(1)**, 27–41.

Cale, L. & Harris, J. (2002) National fitness testing for children – issues, concerns and alternatives, *The British Journal of Teaching Physical Education*, **33(1)**, 32–4.

Cale, L., Harris, J. & Leggett, G. (2002) Making a difference? Lessons learned from a health-related exercise resource, *The Bulletin of Physical Education*, **38(3)**, 145–60.

Capel, S. (2000) Making change in physical education. In Capel, S. & Piotrowski, S. (eds), *Issues in Physical Education*. London: Routledge/Falmer, 221–40.

Corbin, C. B. (2002) Physical activity for everyone: what every physical educator should know about promoting lifelong physical activity, *Journal of Teaching in Physical Education*, **21**, 128–44.

Dale, D., Corbin, C. B. & Cuddihy, T. F. (1988) Can conceptual physical education promote physically active lifestyles? *Pediatric Exercise Science*, **10**, 97–109.

Darling-Hammond, L. (1990) Instructional policy into practice: 'The power of the bottom over the top', *Educational Evaluation and Policy Analysis*, **12**, 233–41.

Davis, S. M., Lambert, L. C., Gomez, Y. & Skipper, B. (1995) Southwest cardiovascular curriculum project: study findings for American Indian elementary students, *Journal of Health Education*, **26** (supplement), S72–81.

DCMS (Department for Culture, Media and Sport) (2001) *A Sporting Future for All. The Government's Plan for Sport*. London: DCMS.

DfES (Department for Education and Skills) (2001) *Specialist Schools Programme: Sports College Applications. A Guide for Schools*. London: DfES.

DfES (Department for Education and Skills) (2002) http://www.standards. dfes. gov.uk/specialistschools/

DfES (Department for Education and Skills) (2003) *Learning Through PE and Sport. A Guide to the Physical Education, School Sport and Club Links Strategy*. London: DfES.

Donnelly, J. E., Jacobsen, D. J., Whatley, J. E. et al. (1996) Nutrition and physical activity program to attenuate obesity and promote physical activity and metabolic fitness in elementary school children, *Obesity Research*, **4**, 229–43.

Dwyer, T., Coonan, W. E., Leitch, D. R., Hetzel, B. S. & Baghurst, R. A. (1983) An investigation of the effects of daily physical activity on the health of primary school students in South Australia, *International Journal of Epidemiology*, **12**, 308–13.

Epstein, L. H., Valoski, A., Wing, R. R. & McCurley, J. (1994) Ten-year outcomes of behavioural family-based treatment for childhood obesity, *Health Psychology*, **13**, 373–83.

Fairclough, S., Stratton, G. & Baldwin, G. (2002) The contribution of secondary school physical education to lifetime physical activity, *European Physical Education Review*, **8(1)**, 69–84.

Fardy, P. S., White, R. E. & Haltiwanger-Schmitz, K. (1996) Coronary disease risk factor reduction and behavior modification in minority adolescents: the PATH program, *Journal of Adolescent Health*, **18**, 247–53.

Fox, K. & Harris, J. (2003) Promoting physical activity through schools. In McKenna, J. & Riddoch, C. (eds), *Perspectives on Health and Exercise*. Basingstoke: Palgrave Macmillan, 181–201.

Goldfine, B. D. & Nahas, M. V. (1993) Incorporating health-fitness concepts in secondary school physical education curricula, *Journal of School Health*, **63(3)**, 142–6.

Gortmaker, S. L., Cheung, L. W., Peterson, K. E. et al. (1999b) Impact of a school-based interdisciplinary intervention on diet and physical activity among urban primary school children: eat well and keep moving, *Archives of Pediatrics and Adolescent Medicine*, **153**, 975–83.

Gortmaker, S. L., Peterson, K., Wiecha, J. et al. (1999a) Reducing obesity via a school-based interdisciplinary intervention among youth: Planet Health, *Archives of Pediatric and Adolescent Medicine*, **153**, 409–18.

Green, K. (2002) Physical education and the 'couch potato society' – part one, *European Journal of Physical Education*, **7(2)**, 95–107.

Harrell, J. S., McMurray, R. G., Bangdiwali, S. I., Frauman, A. C., Gansky, S. A. & Bradley, C. B. (1996) Effects of a school-based intervention to reduce cardio-vascular disease risk factors in elementary-school children: The Cardiovascular Health in Children (CHIC) Study, *J Pediatr*, **128**, 797–805.

Harris, J. (2000) *Health-Related Exercise in the National Curriculum. Key Stages 1 to 4*. Leeds: Human Kinetics.

Harris, J. & Cale, L. (1997) How healthy is school PE? A review of the effectiveness of health-related physical education programmes in schools, *Health Education Journal*, **56**, 84–104.

Harris, J. & Elbourn, J. (1992) Highlighting health related exercise within the National Curriculum – Part Two, *British Journal of Physical Education*, **23(2)**, 5–9.

HEA (Health Education Authority) *Young and Active? Policy Framework for Young People and Health-Enhancing Physical Activity*. London: HEA.

Hendley, K. (2003) High impact of initiative overload? www.sportsteacher.co.uk/features/editorial/sportengland.html

Homel, P. J., Daniels, P., Reid, T. R. & Lawson, J. S. (1981) Results of an experi-mental school-based health development program in Australia, *International Journal of Health Education*, **24**, 263–70.

Hopper, C. A., Gruber, M. B., Munoz, K. D. & Herb, R. A. (1992) Effect of including parents in a school-based exercise and nutrition program for children, *Research Quarterly for Exercise and Sport*, **63**, 315–21.

Ignico, A. A. & Mahon, A. D. (1995) The effects of a physical fitness program on low-fit children, *Research Quarterly for Exercise and Sport*, **66(1)**, 85–90.

Kahn, E. B., Ramsey, L. T., Brownson, R. C., Health, G. W., Howze, E. H. & Powell, K. E. (2002) The effectiveness of interventions to increase physical activity, *American Journal of Preventive Medicine*, **22(4S)**, 73–107.

Kelder, S. H., Perry, C. L. & Klepp, K. I. (1993) Community-wide youth exercise promotion: long-term outcomes of the Minnesota Heart Health Program and the Class of 89 Study, *Journal of School Health*, **63(5)**, 218–23.

Kemper, H. C. G. (1990) Exercise and training in childhood and adolescence. In Torg, J., Welsh, P. & Shephard, R. J. (eds), *Current Therapy in Sports Medicine 2*. Philadelphia, PA: B. C. Decker, 11–17.

Killen, J. D., Telch, M. J., Robinson, T. N., Maccoby, N., Taylor, C. B. & Farquhar, J. W. (1988) Cardiovascular disease risk reduction for tenth graders: a multiple-factor school-based approach, *Journal of the American Medical Association*, **260**, 1728–33.

Kirk, D., Fitzgerald, H., Wang., J. & Biddle, S. (2000) *Towards Girl-Friendly Physical Education: The Nike/ YST Girls in Sport Partnership Project: Final Report*. Institute of Youth Sport: Loughborough University.

Luepker, R. V., Perry, C. L., McKinlay, S. M, Nader, P. R., Parcel, G. S. et al. (1996) Outcomes of a field trial to improve children's dietary patterns and physical activity: The Child and Adolescent Trial for Cardiovascular Health (CATCH), *Journal of the American Medical Association*, **275(10)**, 768–76.

MacConnie, S. E., Gilliam, D. L., Geenen, D. L. & Pels A. E. III (1982) Daily physical activity patterns of prepubertal children involved in a vigorous exercise program, *International Journal of Sports Medicine*, **3**, 202–7.

Manios, Y., Moschandreas, J., Hatzis, C. & Kafatos, A. (1999) Evaluation of a health and nutrition education program in primary school children of Crete over a three-year period, *Preventive Medicine*, **28**, 149–59.

McKenzie, T. L. (2001) Promoting physical activity in youth: focus on middle school environments, *Quest*, **53(3)**, 326–34.

McKenzie, T. L., Nader, P. R., Strikmiller, P. K., Yang, M, Stone, E. J. et al. (1996) School physical education: effect of the Child and Adolescent Trial for Cardiovascular Health, *Preventive Medicine*, **25**, 423–31.

McKenzie, T. L., Sallis, J. F., Kolody, B. & Faucett, F. N. (1997) Long-term effects of a physical education curriculum and staff development work: SPARK, *Research Quarterly for Exercise and Sport*, **68**, 280–91.

Nader, P. R., Sallis, J. F., Patterson, T. L., Abramson, I. S. Rupp, J. W. et al. (1989) A family approach to cardiovascular risk reduction: results from the San Diego Family Health Project, *Health Education Quarterly*, **16**, 229–44.

Nader, P. R., Sellers, D. E., Johnson, C. C., Perry, C. L., Stone, E. J., Cook, K. C. et al. (1996) The effect of adult participation in a school-based family intervention to improve children's diet and physical activity: The Child and Adolescent Trial for Cardiovascular Health, *Preventive Medicine*, **25**, 455–64.

O'Donovan, T. (2002) *The Nike/Youth Sport Trust Girls in Sport Partnership. End of Year Report, December 2002.* Loughborough University: Institute of Youth Sport.

Pangrazi, R. P. (2000) Promoting physical activity for youth, *The ACHPER Healthy Lifestyles Journal*, **47(2)**, 18–21.

Parcel, G. S., Simons-Morton, B., O'Hara, N. M., Baranowski, T. & Wilson, B. (1989) School promotion of healthful diet and physical activity: impact on learning outcomes and self-reported behaviour, *Health Education Quarterly*, **16**, 181–99.

Pate, R. R., Ward, D. S., Felton, G., Saunders, R., Trost, S. G. & Dowda, M. (1997) Effects of a community-based intervention on physical activity and fitness in rural youth, *Medicine and Science in Sports and Exercise*, **29**, S157.

Pate, R., Trost, S., Mullis, R., Sallis, J., Wechsler, H. & Brown, D. (2000) Community interventions to promote proper nutrition and physical activity among youth, *Preventive Medicine*, **31**(supplement), S138–49.

Patrick, K., Sallis, J., Prochaska, J., Lydston, D., Calfas, K., Zabinski, M. et al. (2001) A multi-component program for nutrition and physical activity change in primary care: PACE+ for adolescents, *Archives of Pediatric and Adolescent Medicine*, **155**, 940–6.

Penney, D. & Evans, J. (1999) *Politics, Policy and Practice in Physical Education.* London: E. & F. N. Spon.

Penney, D., Houlihan, B. & Eley, D. (2002) *Specialist Sports Colleges National Monitoring and Evaluation Research Project: First National Survey Report.* Loughborough University: Institute of Youth Sport.

Perry, C. L., Klepp, K. I., Dudovitz, B., Golden, D. & Griffin Smyth, M. (1987) Promoting healthy eating and physical activity patterns among adolescents: a pilot study of 'Slice of Life', *Health Education Quarterly*, **2**, 93–103.

Pieron, M., Cloes, M., Delfosse, C. & Ledent, M. (1996) An investigation of the effects of daily physical education in kindergarten and elementary schools, *European Physical Education Review*, **2(2)**, 116–32.

Resnicow, K., Robinson, T. N. & Frank, E. (1996) Advances and future directions for school-based health promotion research: commentary on the CATCH intervention trial, *Preventive Medicine*, **25**, 378–83.

Richter, K., Harris, K., Paine-Andrews, A., Fawcett, S., Schmid, T. et al. (2000) Measuring the health environment of physical activity and nutrition among youth: a review of the literature and applications for community initiatives, *Preventive Medicine*, **31** (supplement), S98–111.

Robinson, T. N. (1999) Reducing children's television viewing to prevent obesity: a randomised control trial, *Journal of the American Medical Association*, **282**, 1561–7.

Rowland, T. W. (1995) The Horse is Dead; Let's Dismount, *Pediatric Exercise Science*, **7**, 117–20.

Sallis, J. F. (1998) Family and community interventions to promote physical activity in young people. In Biddle, S., Sallis, J. & Cavill, N. (eds), *Young and Active? Young People and Health-Enhancing Physical Activity – Evidence and Implications.* London: HEA, 150–61.

Sallis, J. F., McKenzie, T. L., Alcaraz, J. E., Kolody, B., Faucette, N. & Hovell, M. F. (1997) The effects of a 2-year physical education programme (SPARK) on physical activity and fitness in elementary school students, *American Journal of Public Health*, **87(8)**, 1328–34.

Sallis, J. F., Patrick, K., Frank, E., Pratt, M., Wechsler, H. & Galuska, D. (2000) Interventions in health care settings to promote healthful eating and physical activity in children and adolescents, *Preventive Medicine*, **31** (supplement), S112–20.

Sallis, J. F., Simons-Morton, B. G., Stone, E. J., Corbin, C. B., Epstein, L. H. et al. (1992) Determinants of physical activity in youth, *Medicine and Science in Sports and Exercise*, **24(6)** (supplement), S248–57.

Shephard, R. J. & Lavallee, H. (1993) Impact of enhanced physical education in the prepubescent child: Trois Rivières revisited, *Pediatric Exercise Science*, **5**, 177–89.

Shephard, R. J. & Lavallee, H. (1994) Impact of enhanced physical education on muscle strength of the prepubescent child, *Pediatric Exercise Science*, **6**, 75–87.

Shephard, R. J. & Trudeau, F. (2000) The legacy of physical education: influences on adult lifestyle, *Pediatric Exercise Science*, **12**, 34–50.

Simons-Morton, B. G., Parcel, G. S., Baranowski, T., Forthofer, R. & O'Hara, N. M. (1991) Promoting physical activity and a healthful diet among children: results of a school-based intervention study, *American Journal of Public Health*, **81**, 986–91.

Sparkes, A. (1991) Curriculum change: on gaining a sense of perspective. In Armstrong, N. & Sparkes, A. (eds), *Issues in Physical Education*. London: Cassell, 1–19.

Stone, E. J., McKenzie, T. L., Welk, G. J. & Booth, M. L. (1998) Effects of physical activity interventions in youth: review and synthesis, *American Journal of Preventive Medicine*, **15(4)**, 298–315.

Taggart, A. C., Taggart, J. & Siedentop, D. (1986) Effects of a home-based activity programme: a study with low-fitness elementary school children, *Behaviour Modification*, **10**, 487–507.

Tell, G. S. & Vellar, O. D. (1987) Noncommunicable disease risk factor intervention in Norwegian adolescents: The Oslo Youth Study. In Hetzel, B. & Berenson, G. (eds), *Cardiovascular Risk Factors in Childhood: Epidemiology and Prevention*. Amsterdam: Elsevier Science Publishers, 203–17.

Tinning, R. & Kirk, D. (1991) *Daily Physical Education. Collected Papers on Health Based Physical Education in Australia*. Geelong, Australia: Deakin University Press.

Trudeau, F. Laurencelle, L., Tremblay, J., Rajic, M. & Shephard, R. J. (1998) Follow-up of the Trois Rivières growth and development longitudinal study, *Pediatric Exercise Science*, **10**, 368–77.

Trudeau, F., Laurencelle, L., Tremblay, J., Rajic, M. & Shephard, R. J. (1999) Daily primary school physical education: effects on physical activity during adult life, *Medicine and Science in Sports and Exercise*, **31**, 111–17.

Wechsler, H., Devereaux, R., Davis, M. & Collins, J. (2000) Using the school environment to promote physical activity and healthy eating, *Preventive Medicine*, **31** (supplement), S121–37.

YST (Youth Sport Trust) (2002) www.youthsporttrust.org/yst_schools_ssco.html.

Index

271